W0043560

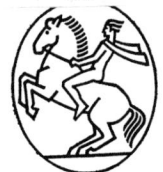

ACTA NEUROCHIRURGICA

SUPPLEMENTUM 31

Ernst Grote

The CNS Control of Glucose Metabolism

SPRINGER-VERLAG

WIEN NEW YORK

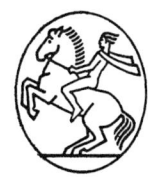

Dr. med. ERNST HEINRICH GROTE

Professor of Neurosurgery
University Clinics Giessen, Federal Republic of Germany

With 95 Figures

Library of Congress Cataloging in Publication Data. Grote, Ernst, 1938—. The CNS control of
glucose metabolism. (Acta neurochirurgica: Supplementum; 31) Bibliography: p. 1. Glucose — Metabolism. 2. Central nervous system. 3. Metabolic regulation. 4. Central nervous system — Diseases — Complications and sequelae. I. Title. II. Series. [DNLM: 1. Central nervous system — Metabolism. 2. Glucose —
Metabolism. W1 AC8661 no. 31 / WL 300 G881c] QP702.G56G76.612'.396.80-26698.

ISSN 0065-1419
ISBN-13:978-3-211-81619-6   e-ISBN-13:978-3-7091-8609-1
DOI: 10.1007/978-3-7091-8609-1

Foreword

In the clinic at Giessen during the last few years there has been an extensive programme of research into the various aspects of lesions of the diencephalon and brain stem and the associated autonomic and metabolic disturbances. As a continuation of this research programme Ernst Grote has investigated the central neuronal and hormonal factors acting on the peripheral regulation of glucose metabolism and their diverse inter-relationships. This research was made possible not only by the availability of well-documented clinical and experimental material with primary and secondary lesions of the hypothalamus and brain stem, but also by the advances in clinical endocrinology and the development of radio-immuno-assays.

By continuous systematic investigation of the basic values and their reaction to stress-tests, as well as to trauma and operation, he has elucidated the basic facts of the central and peripheral mechanisms which are concerned in the regulation of glucose, and also their disturbances.

Of particular significance are his descriptions and interpretations of the characteristic hypothalamic syndromes, as combinations of hyperglycaemia, hyperinsulinaemia and hyperglucagonaemia; different syndromes are produced by lesions at various levels of the brain stem and in central brain death. From this starting point it was possible to develop a rational treatment of this hormonal dysregulation by means of somatostatin.

This work represents the first basic investigation into the central control of glucose metabolism. It has contributed important knowledge about the control of central neuronal and hormonal regulation and dysregulation in the region of the hypothalamus and brain stem. In addition, he has created the prerequisites for future research in the field of energy metabolism.

Giessen, April 1981

HANS WERNER PIA

Contents

1. Introduction

The starting point for the investigations which are presented here, was the clinical observation that a rise of blood sugar can occur in brain diseases and injuries. The extent and duration of this hyperglycaemia was variable and seemed to be related to the clinical severity of the neurological syndrome. In addition the hyperglycaemia was associated with central dysregulation of the various autonomic functions (Pia 1973) such as blood pressure and pulse (Lorenz 1973), respiration (Seeger 1968), temperature (Lausberg 1970), as well as disturbances of the metabolism of water and electrolytes (Wesemann 1973) and the amino-acids (Bauer 1974). This would seem to indicate that the hyperglycaemia is but one part of a general reaction of the organism to particular acute lesions of the brain or is a component of a complete switch over of autonomic function and metabolism in arch to achieve a particular performance. One is frequently able to establish a very close temporal relationship between certain acute brain lesions or complications after neurosurgical interventions and the extent of the hyperglycaemia which develops. The question which arises from this is, whether injury or stimulation of any particular brain structures especially the diencephalon and brain stem are of significance.

Specially directed investigations had shown that marked hyperglycaemia is only rarely accompanied by a ketoacidosis; that even large amounts of exogenous insulin do not definitely influence the level of the blood sugar (Wesemann and Grote 1971, and Pia 1973) and that the loss of glucose through the kidney was sometimes unrelated to the blood sugar level (Wesemann and Grote 1973). The problem from this concerns the precise nature of the disturbance of glucose metabolism observed in cerebral disorders.

The objective of the investigation was

1. To determine which type of hyperglycaemia occurs in the neurosurgical material.

2. To study whether any particular pattern of behaviour of the hyperglycaemia can be related to particular brain lesions or levels of injury.

3. To indicate the mechanisms concerned in the central nervous control of glucose metabolism.

4. To identify the central regulation of the hormones relevant to carbohydrate metabolism and also their dysregulation in relation to the level of the brain lesion.

5. To clarify the pathological significance of hyperglycaemia in diffuse and localized cerebral lesion and hence to develop appropriate lines of treatment.

The investigations were undertaken as a clinical experimental study of patients in the neurosurgical department.

They include:

a) The measurement of blood sugar in a "steady state" and its spontaneous behaviour, as well as the estimation of the hormones which influence it, viz. insulin, glucagon, growth hormone and cortisol in blood and the urinary catecholamines, for several days post-operatively or after injury.

b) The estimation of blood sugar and hormones after deliberate and standardized disturbance of the steady state by an intravenous glucose load.

In certain cases the free fatty acids were determined and the patients stressed by arginine, somatostatin and insulin-hypoglycaemia.

c) The analysis of the glucose utilization by the pharmacokinetic principles introduced by Dost (1968).

d) Statistical evaluation.

2. The Regulation of Glucose Metabolism

2.1. Non-Nervous Regulation

2.1.1. Intrinsic Cell Mechanisms

In the fasting state the level of blood sugar in man is regulated at 60–100 mg%. Glucose breakdown and production run parallel to each other. The breakdown takes place for the most part by glycolysis, the so-called Embden-Meyerhoff chain and to a lesser degree by the pentose-phosphate cycle and the glycuronic acid pathway (Horekker 1967). According to Forster, Holldorf, and Falk (1968) the amount processed by the pentose-phosphate cycle is 2%, although in diabetes mellitus it can rise to 6%. The individual stages of glycolysis facilitate the gradual utilization of the energy which is stored in glucose. Enzymes catalyse the speed of the individual reaction. The fine and intrinsic cellular regulation results from the variations of the speed of reaction, whereby the concentration of the participants in the reaction rapidly modifies the activity of the enzymes. This autoregulation functions independently of nervous control and even in the absence of hormonal activity.

While the glycolytic breakdown is going on in all the organs glucose production takes place in the liver and kidney from gluconeogenesis and glycogenolysis, and from the latter also in the muscles.

Glycogen phosphorylase is controlled in the liver by a cascade mechanism (Mennert and Förster 1970) (Fig. 1) and free glucose is passed into the blood, while after glycogenolysis lactate is formed in the muscles by means of glycolysis which is utilized in the liver for gluconeogenesis (Cori-cycle).

Gluconeogenesis plays a significantly greater role in supplying the organism with glucose than glycogenolysis, as the reserves of glycogen even in a well-nourished man cannot even meet the requirements of glucose for twenty-four hours. After eighteen hours fasting the entire glycogen reserves are exhausted and gluconeogenesis through various preliminary stages remains the only source of glucose. It works through the same metabolic pathways as glycolysis. However, some stages of glycolysis controlled by key-enzymes must be bypassed

1*

because on thermo-dynamic grounds they are irreversible (Walli and Schimassek 1971, Heldt 1972, Soling 1974).

The intrinsic cellular regulation becomes effective through these key enzymes. The building materials for gluconeogenesis are lactate and the "glucoplastic" amino-acids, especially alanine.

In this way the liver represents the centre for glucose homeostasis in the fasting state and it maintains the blood sugar within well defined limits, even after denervation and without any hormonal

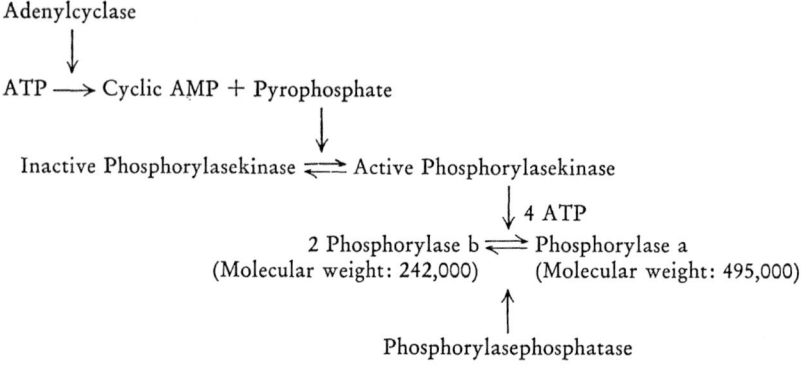

Fig. 1. (After Mehnert and Förster)

control, e.g. it suspends the production of glucose immediately, if glucose is supplied (Soskin and Levine 1952, Leuthardt 1963, Söling 1974). To a certain extent only the kidney is able to contribute to the supply of glucose by neogenesis. According to Holldorf (1974) this proportion can rise to 40% with acidosis, if the kidney has large amounts of NH_4^+ available for counter-regulation. Therefore in acute starvation the liver and kidneys must meet the needs of the organism for glucose, by glycogenolysis and particularly by gluconeogenesis. Their production capacity is estimated at 200 to 300 g/24 hours and the need of the entire organism at 220 g/24 hours (Walli and Schimassek 1971, Knick, Mehnert, and Schoffling 1974). All further energy requirements of the organism are satisfied by free fatty acids and ketone bodies.

According to investigations by Erbslöh (1958) the brain with an average weight of 1,400 g and a circulation of 60 ml/100 g weight uses 80 mg/minute of gulcose, i.e. 115 g/24 hours, while the production of the liver is estimated at 130 mg/minute. Therefore about 60% of the hepatic production is demanded by the brain. Erbslöh (1958) states that the cerebral utilization in various test subjects and in different types of illness is very constant. It remains unchanged not only in diabetic acidosis but also in hyperglycaemia. Only with blood sugar values around 30 mg% is there a reduction in the amount used. This is not dependent on hepatic production, but on the oxidative brain metabolism and this is uninfluenced by sleep and narcosis or by mental and physical strain. It rises only with body temperature and in response to adrenaline. Only after hunger of several days duration is the brain able to utilize ketone bodies. Its glucose requirements fall and the utilization of ketone bodies increases ten- to twenty-fold (Wicklmayr and Dietze 1975).

After a carbohydrate meal and a rise of the blood sugar, mechanisms are brought into action, even without considering the hormonal response, which have as their aim the normalizing of the blood sugar level. Glucose enters more quickly into the body cells, than one would expect from the differences in concentration, but particularly into the muscle and fat cells. The principle of a so-called "facilitated diffusion", i.e. a carrier mechanism, is suggested as the explanation of this phenomenon (Heldt 1972). The liver ceases gluconeogenesis and glycogenolysis and hence its glucose production, and polymerizes the glucose into glycogen. Also in this, rapid changes of activity of the synthesizing enzymes play a decisive part (Mehnert and Forster 1970). The glycolytic breakdown is encouraged, lipolysis is repressed, fatty acids are built up from unused C_2 fragments and neutral fats synthesized (lipogenesis). A further factor in the homeostasis is the glucose excretion by the kidney, whose threshold is subject to diverse humoral and nervous factors (Oberdisse and Paraskevopoulous 1941, Robbers 1946, Abramon and Corvillain 1967).

2.1.2. Hormonal Action

Hormones, as coarse regulators are set over the non-nervous intrinsic cellular fine regulation of the blood sugar. It is only through their action when there are stresses imposed on the glucose metabolism that it is possible to avoid excessive fluctuations of the blood sugar and to confer an optimum speed on the regulation. The hormones develop their activity partly by influencing membrane functions (Levine 1970) and partly through rapidly induced variations in the activity of key enzymes and also by induction, i.e. neoformation, which may take from hours up to days (Holldorf, Forster, and Falk 1968).

Insulin, the only hormone which in physiological concentrations lowers the blood sugar, stands in contradistinction to the diabetogenic hormones, glucagon, growth hormone (HGH), the glucocorticoids and the catecholamines adrenaline and noradrenaline. According to recent investigations by Landgraf, Hörl, Weissmann, and Landgraf-Leurs (1975) one should also include prolactin and in smaller amounts the thyroid hormones and the oestrogens (Mehnert and Schöffling 1974). While insulin represents par excellence the anabolic hormone, its antagonists have predominantly catabolic effects.

2.1.2.1. Insulin

Insulin is present in the beta-cells of the pancreas first of all as proinsulin after biosynthesis from 84 amino-acids. The C-peptide (connecting peptide) is split off from this. Schatz, Hinz, Katsilambros, and Pfeiffer (1973) were able to confirm that 50% of the pro-insulin fraction in man is estimated together with insulin by RIA and even under extreme conditions does not rise above 20% of mU/ml.

The oral glucose stimulus leads to a very much stronger insulin secretion than the intravenous and the beta-cells are stimulated by a whole range of intestinal hormones such as gastrin, secretin, cholecystokynin, pancreozymine (Raptis, Dollinger, Schlegel, Nadjafi 1975), enteroglycagon, GIP (gastric inhibiting polypeptide) motilin and incretin (Creutzfeldt 1974). In this connexion Unger and Eisentraut speak about the enteroinsulin axis.

Aminoacids and fatty acids can also promote the secretion of insulin (Pfeiffer 1971, Fussgänger, Hinz, Raptis, Schleyer, and Straub 1971). Simultaneously with the rise in insulin, the glucagon which is produced by the alpha-cells of the pancreas falls. Samols has been able to confirm this mechanism on the isolated perfused dogs pancreas (Fig. 2).

According to Samols (1975) the pancreatic glucagon is an important stimulator of insulin secretion whereas insulin functions as an inhibitor of glucagon secretion. According to Cerasi and Luft (1967) the normal insulin response to glucose, in healthy subjects can vary considerably (low and high responders). The action of insulin was ascertained on a number of tissues including its effect on the brain metabolism (Gottstein and Heldt 1967). However it is of quantitative significance for muscle, fat and liver cells. The mechanism of action in the muscle and fat cells consists of the encouragement of the membrane transport of sugar and amino-acids, in the stimulation of glycogen, protein and triglyceride synthesis in muscle, fat and liver cells and in the inhibition of lipolysis, proteolysis and gluconeogenesis (Mehnert and Schöffling 1974). The cyclic AMP system, the "second messenger", acts as the mediator for the rapid effects of insulin on the different key enzymes (Sutherland and

Robinson 1969). Consequently all the individual actions of insulin work for the storage and the preservation of energy, *i.e.* anabolism (Fig. 3).

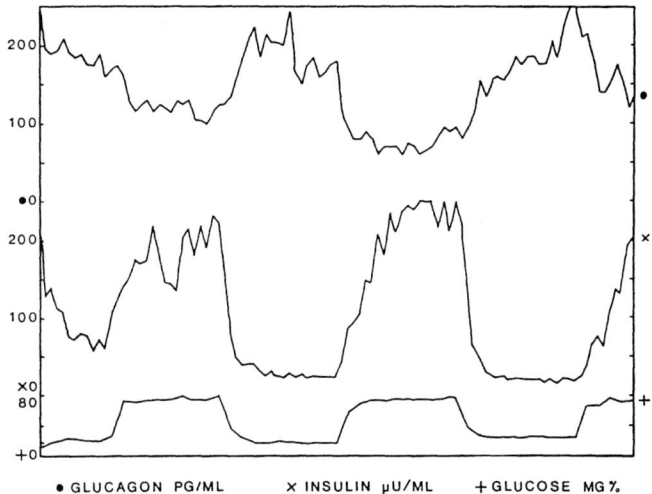

● GLUCAGON PG/ML   ✗ INSULIN μU/ML   + GLUCOSE MG %

Fig. 2. Effect of low and normal glucose on glucagon and insulin secretion. (E. Samols and J. Harrison, personal communication)

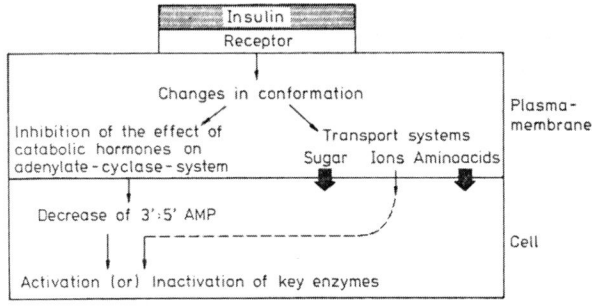

Fig. 3. (From Mehnert and Schöffling 1974)

In connexion with the facilitation of the transport of glucose into the muscle and fat cells, the different actions lead to a lowering of the blood sugar level so that the membrane transport represents the speed limiting factor in carbohydrate metabolism. The glucose assimilation which can be measured by pharmacokinetic investigations, is significantly influenced by the concentration of free fatty acids which, if at a high level, are preferentially utilized by the muscle and fat cells. Glycolysis is repressed, the assimilation is reduced and a varying degree of insulin resistance is produced. The effect of the insulin on the glucose metabolism shows only one of its principle functions. A more important influence on the metabolism of fat is the inhibition of lipolysis.

After a single intravenous glucose load there is a production of insulin within the first two minutes. With continuous glucose stimulation a second insulin peak appears after 30 to 45 minutes (Fig. 4).

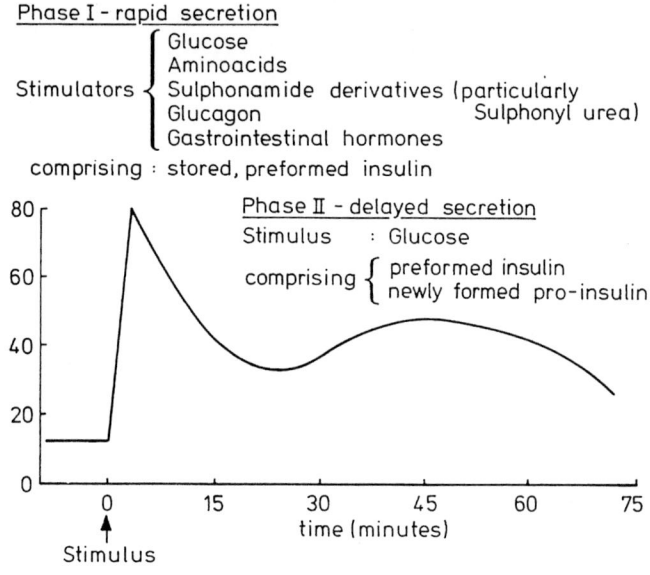

Fig. 4. (From Mehnert and Schöffling 1974)

It is the absolute or relative deficiency of insulin or, expressed in a different way, the disproportion between insulin requirements and production which can be looked on as the pathogenetic characteristic of diabetes mellitus (Pfeiffer 1969, Mehnert and Förster 1970, Mehnert and Schöffling 1974). This disproportion is shown very obviously in the case of diabetes associated with overweight (Pfeiffer 1973). In diabetes four different disturbances of insulin secretion are described (Grabner 1974).

2.1.2.2. Glucagon

Unger and Faloona 1971, Unger, Aguilar-Parade, Muller, and Eisentraut 1970, Unger 1975, and Samols 1975 in discussing the deficiency of insulin have stressed the role of glucagon in the pathophysiology of diabetes mellitus and in this connexion have pointed out that in animal experiments after removal of the intestine and pancreas, and hence the intestinal cells which produce enteroglucagon, the hyperglycaemia remains slight and acidosis does not develop. Also after administration of the hypothalamic "hormone" somatostatin, which inhibits the secretion of growth hormone, insulin and glucagon, the pancreatectomized animal does not lapse into a diabetic coma. Glucagon represents one of the important antagonists of insulin. A glucagon-like substance whose identity with pancreatic glucagon is still under discussion is secreted by certain cells in the small intestine (Mehnert and Schöffling 1974). The action of glucagon on glycogenolysis and gluconeogenesis takes place within seconds. With only a short half life of 5 to 10 minutes the action on glycogenolysis which is mediated through the cyclic AMP system disappears within minutes, while after a single dose gluconeogenesis is stimulated for periods of up to an hour (Sokal 1966). Walli and Schimassek (1971) as well as Sokal, Sarcione, and Henderson (1964) and Sarcione, Sokal, and Gerszi (1960) were able to show that its effects on glycogenolysis occurs at physiological concentrations. Unphysiological doses of adrenaline 10^3 M higher must be used to achieve a comparable effect.

According to Unger and Faloona (1971) the relative molar concentrations of insulin and glucagon in the portal venous blood determine, to what extent energy is stored in the form of carbohydrate, fat and protein or is made available in the periphery as glucose, free fatty acids and amino-acids. Unger (1971, 1972) has thus introduced the concept of the insulin-glucagon quotient, which represents a figure for describing the metabolic situation at any particular time. In starvation it can fall to a value of 0.3 to 0.4 showing the state of catabolism and after a carbohydrate meal it can rise to 16–36 and thereby give a hint as to the anabolic state of the metabolism. The authors regard the islets of Langerhans as a "push-pull-organ".

While glucagon promotes the secretion of insulin and, vice versa, insulin suppresses the secretion of glucagon (Samols 1975, Unger 1975), both hormones produce a rise with an amino-acids load, e.g. arginine and a fall with somatostatin and diazoxide (Samols 1975), and that regardless of the height of the blood sugar. Hautecouverture, Basdevant, Slama, and Tchobroutsky had established in 1975 that the insulin secretion produced by arginine and glucagon was significantly lower in both sexes in the afternoon than in the morning, so that an endogenous rhythm of the beta-cells was discussed. After the somatostatin produced inhibition of the initial insulin peak after glucose the K-value became pathological (Alberti et al. 1973).

2.1.2.3. Glucocorticoids

In contrast to glucagon and the catecholamines the glucocorticoids do not show their action on the carbohydrate metabolism immediately. They lead rather to an induction of enzymes for gluconeogenesis and, by means of proteolysis and the making available of amino-acids, to stimulation of gluconeogenesis. According to Holldorf (1974) the glucocorticoids, especially cortisol, are absolutely essential for gluconeogenesis from amino-acids, as without cortisol no proteolysis takes place in muscle. This explains the often threatening hypoglycaemia of Addison's disease. Cortisol encourages lipolysis, the increase in free fatty acids leads to inhibition of glucose utilization in the muscle cells and thereby leads to an impairment of glucose assimilation (Tausk 1973), to hyperinsulinism, to relative insulin sensitivity and, by depletion of the pancreatic reserves, to steroid diabetes (Mehnert and Schöffling 1974).

2.1.2.4. Growth Hormone (HGH)

Growth hormone, also, does not exert a speedy, but a prolonged effect on the carbohydrate mechanism. Its secretion from the anterior lobe of the pituitary through the action of the GHRF (growth hormone releasing factor) has been confirmed; this originates from the ventro-medial nucleus of the hypothalamus (Krulich 1974). Its stimulation leads to a rise, and its destruction to a fall, in the amount of growth hormone (Frohman, Bernardis, and Kant 1968). Stimulation or coagulation in the lateral hypothalamus or on the cortex does not produce any change in the growth hormone. The GHIF (growth hormone inhibiting factor) somatostatin was found in the anterior hypothalamus and simultaneously inhibits the secretion of TSH, glucagon and insulin. According to Yalow and Berson (1971) the strongest stimulus to growth hormone secretion is hypoglycaemia. After the administration of glucose the growth hormone level falls. Other potent stimuli are amino-acids, especially arginine, as well as emotional and psychological factors, toxins, physical activity and other situations leading to stress. The rise of the growth hormone produced by these stimuli is contingent on an intact hypothalamo-pituitary system.

The action of the growth hormone (HGH) on the carbohydrate metabolism is rather indirect according to Ditschuneit (1974). First of all the combustion of fatty acids is increased, and hence lipolysis as well; the free fatty acids in their turn impair the utilization of glucose. In addition to this the phosphorylation of glucose is inhibited. Amino-acids are spared at the cost of free fatty acids and protein synthesized so that we find here a synergism with the anabolic effect of insulin. Which of the metabolic processes of the growth hormone is mediated through the sulphation factor, or somatomedin or the Nsilas, and if any relationship exists between these three principles, is still under discussion at present.

Cushing had already noted that about 25% of patients with acromegaly showed a diabetic metabolic disturbance. In Tönnis' material the figure given was 22.5%. Houssay and Biasotti (1931, 1932) were able to demonstrate the diabetogenic effect of pituitary extract and to mitigate and partly abolish the manifestations of diabetes by hypophysectomy.

A direct action of growth hormone on the beta-cells was also debated (Kracht 1953). According to Pfeiffer no significant change of carbohydrate metabolism can be observed immediately after adminisation of growth hormone, however after administration for twelve days the output of insulin in response to glucose is cut down, so that one may assume a direct effect on the beta-cells. Ditschuneit (1974), Sirek, Hotta, and Sirek (1971) immediately after giving growth hormone found no evidence for a stimulation of insulin production. Lipolysis only occurred after hours. The relationships between growth hormone and diabetes or insulin have been discussed in detail by Pfeiffer (1965), Luft and Cerasi (1965), Rabinowitz, Merimee, and Burgess (1966), and Luft and Cerasi (1967). On the other hand acute effects from higher doses of growth hormone were pointed out by Adamson, Cerasi, and Wahren (1975). The basal insulin level was lowered by 10 to 20% while stimulation with glucose, tolbutamide and glucagon yielded up to 40% less insulin response. Also, the glucose tolerance was lowered. Insulin-like effects were shown in the slight fall of the basal glucose level and in the decrease in glucose output by the liver. Thus, it is only with a sustained raised level of growth hormones that diabetes appears and then only if the pancreas is no longer in a position to compensate for the diverse effects of growth hormone by increased production of insulin.

2.2. Central Nervous Regulation

Glucose metabolism is subject to diverse regulation mechanisms. At cellular level, fine regulation and control results from changes in the enzyme activity. This control undergoes a quantitative extension, acceleration of the speed of reaction and an optimizing through the action of hormones. These are for the most part secreted and inhibited without the necessity of any neural control. Isolated islets on stimulation with glucose will secrete insulin and an isolated pancreas with glucopaenia will secrete glucagon. A denervated liver produces glucose and adjusts its production according to the needs of the organism. However, in the presence of impending hypo-glycaemia the resulting secretion of growth hormone and ACTH, *i.e.* cortisol and other corticoids, is closely dependent on the structural integrity and function of central nervous structures. The acute dependence of the oxidative brain metabolism on a continuous supply of glucose implies supplementary protective mechanisms not only against, hypoglycaemia but also against the excessive action of peripheral hormones.

The function of the central nervous system in metabolism is not confined to ensuring its own energy requirements with glucose, but consists in the integrated adjustment of metabolism to a particular task and the consequent indispensible coordination of metabolic per-formance. This function is demonstrated very clearly by an experiment of Westerman and Stock (1969) (Fig. 5). Autoregulation and reciprocal influencing of glucose and fatty acids leads in starvation to a rise of free fatty acids and a fall of glucose; after giving glucose the free fatty acids were immediately reversed and their serum concentration fell. The behaviour of this glucose-fatty acid cycle consequently shows a mirror-image pattern with its reaction partner.

On the contrary under cold stress glucose and free fatty acids show a simultaneous rise in the same direction with the aim of making energy available in the struggle against cold (Fig. 6). It has been confirmed by removal of the adrenal medulla and also by sympathectomy, that this synchronous regulation is mediated through the nervous system and subsequently by adrenaline. In such cases glucose and free fatty acids do not rise and the body temperature falls. By giving adrenaline the original pattern of the reaction if restored. The "normal" mirror like influence on free fatty acids and glucose by the nervous system and adrenaline is overridden in the direction of the urgent, essential demand of the body, viz. the supply of energy.

This functional adjustment to a specific metabolic target through the effect of the nervous system was also stressed by Himms-Hagen (1967, 1972). The central stimulation of the sympathetic which arises as a result of the hypoglycaemia, leads to an increase of the "releasing hormones" for ACTH and growth hormone, and in ad-dition to mobilization of glucagon, by the neural pathways, via the adrenal medulla and the secretion of adrenaline. The resulting rise in blood sugar, without the participation by the nervous system, leads to production of insulin and thereby once again to storage of glucose as glycogen and to its consumption in muscle and fat cells.

In this case the effect of the sympathetic stimulation and the supply of glucose would be very brief and could not ensure the nutrition of the brain. However the resulting inhibition of glucose-induced insulin secretion determined by neural factors and catecholamines, simultaneous with the stimulation of the adrenal medulla, hinders the output of insulin (see page 50). It thus happens that the mobilized glucose

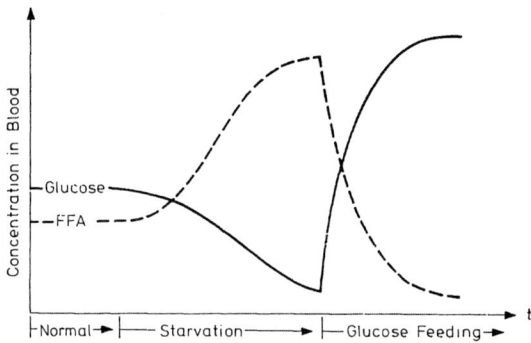

Fig. 5. (After Westerman and Stock 1969)

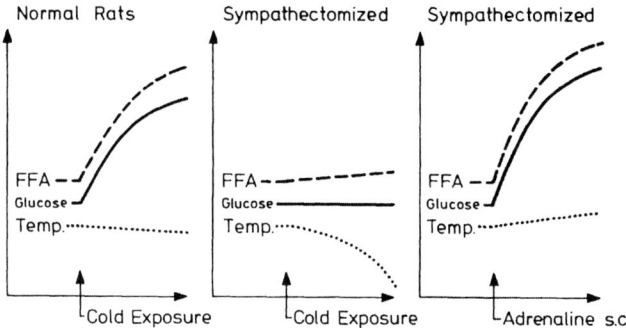

Fig. 6. (After Westerman and Stock 1969)

is not transported to the muscle and fat cells, for without insulin, these are scarcely able to take up glucose. Consequently the mobilized glucose actually remains available to the brain which is threatened by hypoglycaemia, especially as the fatty acids simultaneously raised because of the sympathetic action, also impair the peripheral utilization of glucose. Also, in this example there are several organ system connected together by means of the nervous system with the object of ensuring an efficient control of metabolism. The central nervous system makes use of neural and neurohormonal mechanisms for the safeguarding of its integrative functions. The purpose of this two-pronged flow of information lies on the one hand in the enhanced security of the regulation should there be a failure in one of the mechanisms; on the other hand, different peripheral effectors are employed. The neural transmission of information is effective exclusively through the intrinsic cellular enzyme regulation. Very essential are the variable kinetics. Through the neural pathways the effect is very rapid and is attained within seconds to minutes, however it does not persist for long. Hormones exert their action within minutes, but usually in hours or even days.

2.2.1. Neural Regulation

2.2.1.1. Early Experimental Findings in Animals

Since the account by Claude Bernard (1849) of his "Picqûre", numerous later workers have studied the influence of the nervous system on carbohydrate metabolism and as a consequence have undertaken most diverse experiments. The results have at times been contradictory and have also been interpreted differently. Bernard had sited his "sugar centre" in the medulla oblongata, in the wall of the fourth ventricle between the points of origin of the acoustic and the vagus nerves. Later authors have explained the hyperglycaemia not by the destruction of a centre, but by stimulation of the conduction pathways. Stewart and Rogoff (1918) working with rabbits were regularly able to bring about hyperglycaemia by puncture near the midline at the level of the calamus scriptorius. This also developed after adrenalectomy, so that a direct neural stimulus of the liver cells was regarded as the decisive factor. It was also clear that for the stimulation to be successful a normal content of liver glycogen was a prerequisite. Mellanby in 1920 had seen very marked hyperglycaemia after infarction of a hemisphere and subsequent decerebration. After total brain infarction the blood sugar fell to normal values. It could not be raised again by a subsequent operation or by giving an anaesthetic. Mellanby had assumed the existence of a sugar centre in the brain stem, which after the failure of higher brain regions was no longer controlled and on the other hand could still be stimulated by peripheral afferents. An analogy with the decerebrate rigidity of Sherrington was seen.

Donhoffer and McLeod (1932) have demonstrated by systematic investigations that the piqure hyperglycaemia is delayed by narcosis with amytal or luminal. The authors have made mid-brain lesions ("decerebration") in rabbits at four different levels (Fig. 7). Only by a lesion at level "III", *i.e.* the pons, was a marked hyperglycaemia regularly found, while transverse lesions at the other levels only inconstantly produced an elevation of blood sugar.

Provided that there is no anaesthesia and also a normal glycogen content in the liver, hyperglycaemia can be produced regularly by piqure of the vestibular nucleus. Glycogenolysis and gluconeogenesis were regarded as responsible for the hyperglycaemia. After adrenalectomy hyperglycaemia only appeared if there was a lot of glycogen in the liver.

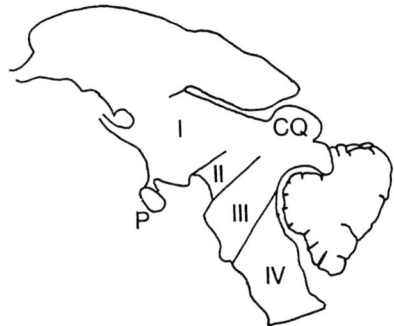

Fig. 7. (After Donhoffer and McLeod 1932)

Hyperglycaemia and pathological glucose tolerance tests were observed in rats after sections through the pons or midbrain (Anderson and Haymaker 1952).

In dogs experimental transverse lesions in the hypothalamus at the level of the optic chiasm had produced sustained hyperglycaemia (d'Amour and Keller 1931). Bilateral stereotactic electrolytic lesions in the hypothalamus of cats produced in 42 out of 55 instances several days sustained elevation of the blood sugar levels (Harris and Ingram 1935). They were not able to establish any relationship between hyperglycaemia and definite regions of the hypothalamus. Not only vago-insulin but also sympathetico-adrenal reactions were described by Anand and Dua (1953) after stimulation of permanently implanted hypothalamic electrodes. Gellhorn (1941) had recorded a fall of blood sugar by stimulation of the hypothalamus after adrenalectomy or high cervical cord section, and this failed to appear after vagotomy.

Grafe (1935) and Strieck (1935) have assumed that important influences emanate from the hypothalamus, without necessarily postulating a "sugar centre"; hyperglycaemia has been observed after stimulation of the stellate ganglion (Davis, Cleveland, and Ingram 1935, and Reiss 1950).

2.2.1.2. "Neurotraumatic" Diabetes

While these authors regard central hyperglycaemia as a transient disturbance and "central diabetes" as a rarity, Vonderrahe (1937) and Morgan et al. (1937) were discussing changes in the hypothalamus (nucleus paraventricularis) as a possible cause of diabetes mellitus. Strieck (1938) reported on a persistent hyperglycaemia in a dog, produced by infiltration of the hypothalamus with silver nitrate. The animal was followed for two months until its death, and at autopsy there were no pathological findings in the pancreas. Veil and Sturm (1942) on the basis of 40 observations of brain injuries and other lesions have advanced the theory that diabetes mellitus is a neurological symptom; consequently it always develops secondarily and as a sequal to a brain disorder, in the setting of a diencephalosis, in the course of which pancreas and liver only play a minor role. In 1944 Falta had noticed the relationships between diabetes mellitus and hypothalamic disorders, but he indicated nevertheless that there are many grave diencephalic lesions, without any evidence of a disturbance of carbohydrate metabolism. Wedler (1948) is opposed to the concept of "neurotraumatic diabetes". Forty-five acutely injured with retained metal fragments in various parts of the diencephalon and brain stem were examined. Signs of severe neurological deficit and autonomic disturbances of water and energy metabolism tended to improve. In a total of 2,000 brain injuries no permanent diabetes could be found. Zülch (1950) in his report on circumscribed injuries of the diencephalon wrote that autonomic disturbances develop immediately after the injury and mostly disappear after some time, and a genuine ("medical") internal disorder does not develop. Orthner (1955) and Erbslöh (1958) contradict the concept of "neural pathology". Hügler (1950) and Pausch (1951) had indeed accepted a functional disturbance of the islets of Langerhans as essential for the development of diabetes mellitus, but they advocate the view that a more severe psychic shock or a hypothalamic disturbance associated with a corresponding predisposition can lead to diabetes mellitus. Shull and Meyer (1956) point out nevertheless that the so-called neurogenic hyperglycaemia produced by stimulation such as the piqure, last only for a few hours up to two days, while hypothalamic lesions can lead to hyperglycaemia lasting days or weeks. *The First International Neuroautonomic Symposium* in Florence was concerned with the main topic of autonomic neural influences on sugar metabolism (Anderson, Suronini, Critchley, Gellhorn, Lopez, Prieto, Lunedei, de Morsier, and Sturm 1954). Contradictory results and theories were reported. Lubken (1960) regards the neuroautonomic influence as an additional protective mechanism, while the hormonal regulation takes place even without any neural mechanisms. Bertram and Otto (1963) actually stress the hormonal and nervous connexion between the diencephalon and all organ systems; they advocate the view however that in general even severe destructive central lesions do not cause any peripheral disease. The defective central control can only lead to disease, when the periphery is no longer able to compensate for it. Diabetes mellitus may be explained in every case by an absolute or relative deficiency of insulin.

2.2.1.3. Diencephalic Structures and Organization of the Autonomic Nervous System. Results of Stimulation and Ablation Experiments

The basic theoretical and anatomical requirements for an intensive experimental investigation of the neural influence of the hypothalamus on carbohydrate metabolism and the hormones which control it, have been given in the papers of Hess (1948). The stepwise organization of the autonomic nervous system and the demarcation of a dynamogenic and an endophylactic-trophotropic zone in the hypothalamus have stimulated the research in this field. The brain stem was defined not in terms of anatomy, but as the dynamic starting point for the complex mutual interaction of several organ system. As a result Hess has pointed out, that peripheral functions and a resting tonus in the sympathetic and parasympathetic are not lost and in the presence of central paralysis these archaic mechanisms once again come into play. The neuronal connexious within the hypothalamus itself and with its surroundings have been described and discussed by Penfield (1934), Raisman (1966), Ganon (1966), Lammers (1969) and particularly by Ban (1966). According to his own and experimental work by Kourotsu his septo-preoptico-hypothalamic system (Fig. 8) consists firstly of a parasympathetic area A, composed of the septal region of the periventricular zone and the medial mamillary nucleus and secondly of a parasympathetic area C, which is connected rostrally to the septal region and towards the posterior part consists of the lateral hypothalamic nucleus. The sympathetic zone B consists of the medial preoptic field, the entire group of medial nuclei and the mamillary nuclei. By special anatomical experimental techniques, descending fibres from the B-zone have been traced through the central grey matter down to the level of the superior colliculi. By stimulation and ablation experiments Ban has been able

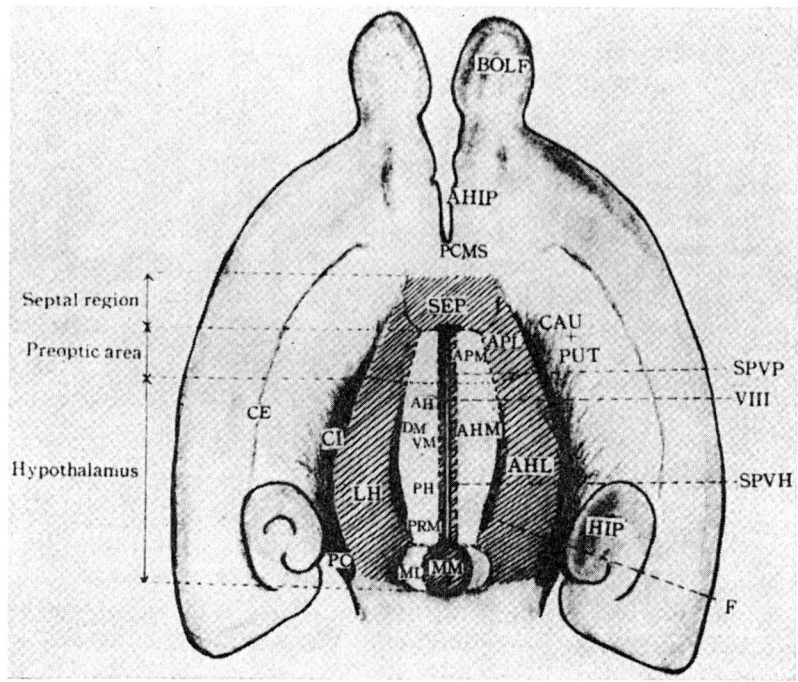

Fig. 8. Septo-preoptico-hypothalamic system (SPH system) of the rabbit brain. Horizontal section through the septal region, preoptic area and hypothalamus. Area parasympathica A consisting of the septal region (*SEP*), preoptic periventricular stratum (*SPVP*), hypothalamic periventricular stratum (*SPVH*) and medial mamillary nucleus (*MM*), and area parasympathica C consisting of the septal region, lateral preoptic area (*APL*) and lateral hypothalamic area (*AHL*) are marked by oblique lines. Areas A and C unite in the septal region. The medial preoptic area (*APM*), medial hypothalamicarea (*AHM*) and lateral mamillary nucleus (*ML*) belong to area sympathica B. *AH* anterior hypothalamic nucleus, *AHIP* anterior continuation of the hippocampus, *BOLF* bulbus olfactorius, *CAU* caudate nucleus. *CE* external capsule, *CI* internal capsule, *DM* dorsomedial hypothalamic nucleus. *F* fornix, *HIP* hippocampus, *PH* posterior hypothalamic nucleus, *PC* cerebral peduncle, *PCMS* precommissural portion of the septum, *PRM* premamillary nucleus, *PUT* putamen, *VM* ventromedial hypothalamic nucleus

to verify the neuronal connexion of the medial B-zone right as far as the intermedio-lateral column of the cervical spinal cord. Beattie, Brow, and Long were successful in proving these connexions as early as 1930. Moreover, of greater significance is the fact of repeated neuronal ablations, some at the level of the superior colliculus, and others at the level of the vestibular nucleus (Ban 1966).

In 1957 Kourotsu, after ventro-medial stimulation was able to produce an increase in the number of beta-cells in the pancreas and a reduction in number after stimulation of the lateral part of the thalamus. With ventro-medial stimulation the vacuole formation in the beta-cells increased and after lateral stimulation it decreased again, as there was an outflow of secretion. These results can be obtained even after preliminary adrenalectomy.

Kaneto *et al.* (1965) were able to prevent the rise of "insulin-like activity" after adrenalectomy and hypophysectomy, by stimulation of the dorsal and rostral portion of the cingulate gyrus, whereas stimulation of other parts of the cingulate gyrus produced no effect. After bilateral electrolytic lesions of the ventro-medial nucleus in rats, Frohman and Bernadis (1968) have observed a decrease of the growth hormone and hyperglycaemia with hyperinsulinaemia. Also, Booth *et al.* (1969) found a rise in blood sugar after ventro-medial stimulation, which was no longer apparent after bilateral adrenal-ectomy. Occasionally after stereotactic operations for pain in the posterior part of B-zone as well as ergotropic reactions there was also found to be a slight rise in blood sugar, an excessive rise of growth hormone and an even more marked rise of free fatty acids (Sano, Mayanagi, Sekino, Ogashiva, and Ishijima 1970). After ventro-medial hypothalamic stimulation Frohman and Bernadis (1971) had observed a normal rate of disappearance of C^{14} labelled glucose in hyperglycaemia. The initial rise of glucose after stimulation was not prevented by adrenalectomy, but however the later was. In spite of the increase of blood sugar the secretion led to a rise of glucagon and that even after adrenalectomy, so that the direct neural stimulus of the alpha-cells of the pancreas must be decisive. The region of the ventro-medial hypothalamus from which the reaction described was obtained, coincides with the B-zone of Ban. The authors were able to show (1972) that bilateral ventro-medial hypothalamic lesions in rats lead to increases in the reactive insulin levels. As the utilization of C^{14} labelled glucose was as high as in the control group, a periph-eral insulin resistence could not be accepted as the cause of the high insulin levels. Frohman (1975) showed in his experiments that the fine and immediate regulation took place directly through the ventro-medial hypothalamic nuclei, the central grey matter, the floor of the fourth ventricle, through the spinal cord, the splanchnic nerve and the liver cells, while the hormonal regulation sustains the initial neural effect, in this instance by inhibition of the insulin secretion through adrenaline, through maintenance of glycogenolysis and pro-motion of gluconeogenesis by the glucagon. Under normal conditions the sympathetic, *i.e.* the ventro-medial nucleus should inhibit the parasympathetic system, *i.e.* the lateral hypothalamic nucleus.

2.2.1.4. Neural Influences on the Liver Cells, on Glycogenolysis and Glycogen Synthesis

The neural, non-hormonal control of the brain on the liver cells has been pointed out by Erbslöh (1958) on the basis of his clinical observations. In the literature there have been reports of an immediate hepatic jaundice after a shock and also of a transitory hepatogenetic glycosuria occurring as a symptom of mental diseases. Erbslöh has summarized the physiological relationship between brain and liver in three basic statements:

1. Significant central nervous regulating mechanisms exist for the liver.

2. There are indispensible mechanisms in the liver for maintaining the undisturbed activity of the brain.

3. A special co-operation exists between the two organs with regard to their metabolism and vulnerability.

The direct contact of unmyelinated nerve fibres with the surface membranes of the liver cells was shown with the electron microscope by Yamada (1965). Shimizu and Fukuda (1964), and Shimizu, Fukuda, and Ban (1966) have observed hyperglycaemia after ventro-medial stimulation of the hypothalamus. Simultaneously the liver glycogen fell. After stimulation of the splanchnic nerve and of the ventro-medial nuclei the authors have recorded a three-fold rise in the activity of the enzymes glycogenphosphorylase and glucose-6-phosphatase. This effect survived intact after adrenalectomy and pancreatectomy. It was not assumed that glucagon or adrenaline played any part in this. By direct stimulation of the left vagus nerve the total activity of glycogen synthetase was markedly raised (Shimazu 1967). This effect was abolished by simultaneous stimulation of the splanchnic nerve. Conversely the rise of activity of phosphorylase-A after splanchnic stimulation was prevented by simultaneous stimulation of the vagus nerve. This neural regulation of the glycogen metabolism which is independent of the pancreas and adrenals begins ten seconds after stimulation and stops five minutes later (Shimazu 1968). While an increase of activity not only of phosphorylase-A but also of glucose-6-phosphatase appears within seconds after stimulation of the sympathetic, the effect of adrenaline occurs only after minutes and is continued to a rise in activity of phosphorylase-A (Shimazu 1968). It maintains the initial neural effect. The blocking of beta-adrenergic receptors can prevent the action of the catecholamines, but not that of sympathetic stimulations.

Edwards and Silver (1970) have reported on the findings in adrenalectomized calves. After splanchnic stimulation there was hyperglycaemia and a decrease in glycogen. Pancreatectomy did not have any further influence on this effect. Also a humoral factor as mediator was excluded, as the reinfusion of hepatic venous blood produced no tendency towards hyperglycaemia. After partial denervation of the liver, neither the hyperglycaemia response, not the fall of glycogen was any longer detectable. Exton, Robinson, Sutherland, and Park (1971) hold the view that the neural, as well as the hormonal influence on the enzymes is effective through the mediation of the cyclic AMP system.

2.2.1.5. Neural Stimulation of the Adrenal Medulla and the Role of Catecholamines

The adrenal medulla receives its neural impulses through preganglionic fibres from the splanchnic nerve. Boehm and Hoffman had established in 1878 that cats retain their carbohydrate reserves after section of the upper cervical cord and die of hypothermia, whereas if they are mechanically restrained carbohydrates are consumed. Asphyxia and painful stimuli increase the secretion of the adrenal medulla (Cannon and Hoskins 1911). Cannon, McIver, and Bliss (1924) have declared that the strongest stimulus for the secretion of the adrenal medulla is hypoglycaemia. Under laboratory conditions bilateral sympathectomy in cats produces no effect whatsoever and only after stresses such as cold, mechanical restraint and struggling was their evidence of hypothermia and a failure of rise of blood pressure and blood sugar (Cannon, Newton, Bright, Menkin, and Moore 1929). The authors are convinced from their investigations about the significance of the sympathetic nervous system for the flight and combat reaction.

Electrical stimulation of the hypothalamus increases the secretion of the adrenal medulla, particularly the adrenaline fraction (Brücke, Kaindl, and Mayer 1952). The resting secretion of adrenaline and noradrenaline can be reduced by systemic administration of glucose; and it falls still further after a denervation of the adrenals (Duner 1953). After this, elevation of the blood sugar has no further effect on the catecholamine secretion. Also after isolated perfusion of the head of the experimental animal and administration of glucose in the region of the hypothalamus, the catecholamine excretion falls. A rise of glucose in the region of the hypothalamus reduced the neural stimulation of the adrenal medulla and, at the same time, the secretion of "releasing hormone" for the growth hormone and ACTH (see also under "Neurohumoral regulation"). Zunz and la Barre (1927) on the basis of their experiments with crossed circulation had concluded that there was a central region sensitive to glucose. Himsworth

(1970) was able to report on the hypothalamic control of adrenal secretion in the absence of available glucose, after infiltration of the hypothalamus with lignocaine.

The action of adrenaline on the carbohydrate metabolism had already been recognized in 1928 by Cori and Cori. It consists, according to Himms-Hagan (1967, 1972) in the encouragement of gluconeogenesis from lactate and amino-acids and of glycogenolysis in liver and muscle, in the simultaneous provision of free fatty acids and, with that, a reduced utilization of glucose, in the raising of the total consumption and in the so-called calorigenic effect. Furthermore, as is still to be discussed, the insulin secretion is inhibited by the catecholamines and hence the utilization of the mobilized glucose by muscle and fat cells is prevented. The sympathetic-adrenaline system is activated by heat and cold, injuries, emotional and physical stress, reduction of blood pressure, lack of oxygen, awakening from hibernation and particularly by hypoglycaemia (Himms-Hagen 1972). The effect on metabolism by the catecholamines and their pharmacological control has been discussed in detail by Senft (1967), Senft, Sitt, Losert, Schultz, and Hoffman (1968, Westermann and Stock (1969) and also by Himms-Hagen (1962). On account of the general effect of various receptor blockers, any particular experimental results should only be interpreted with considerable reserve.

Rosenberg and Di Stefano (1962) and Ezdini, Javid, Owens, and Sokal (1968) have investigated the action of infused adrenaline on the metabolism in various lesions of the nervous system. They found that after transection of the upper cervical cord or medulla oblongata below the fourth ventricle, the effect was abolished whereas the metabolic effect of adrenaline after transection between the colliculi corresponded with that in control animals. It is postulated that an "intact" midbrain is the prerequisite for the metabolic action of adrenaline.

2.2.1.6. Nerve Supply to the Cells of the Islets of Langerhans

The nerve supply of the pancreas and the islets of Langerhans has been studied in various species by Gentes (1902), Pensa (1905), Feyrter (1954), Esterhuizen and Lever (1961), Winborn (1963), and Lange (1965), as well as more recently by Kobayashi (1966), Leggo (1967), Watari (1968), Koba-Yashi and Fujita (1969), and Schorr and Blum (1970). Esterhuizen, Spriggs, and Lever (1968) found invaginated unmedullated axons on the surface of alpha- and beta-cells in the cats pancreas. Pharmacological investigations revealed the existence not only of cholinergic but also of adrenergic fibres in the alpha- and beta-cells. Findlay et al. (1964) were able to confirm these findings in rabbits and to demonstrate an abrupt rise of insulin after stimulation of a branch of the dorsal vagus nerve. Kern, Hoffman, and Kern (1971) described the abundant nerve cells supplying the islet cells—the so-called neuro-insular complex, which represents a common functional unit consisting of the ganglion and the islet-cells. Kern and Grube produced in 1972 a comparative study of the innervation in various species. Munger (1972) was consistently able to identify alpha-cells in close relationship to the autonomic fibres and, with the electron microscope, to detect the so-called neuro-insular complex in various species of animals.

2.2.1.7. Neural Control of Glucagon Secretion

The functional significance of the nerve supply of the islet cells becomes evident from the results of experimental research on the neurogenic secretion of glucagon and insulin. After electrical stimulation of the splanchnic nerve the secretion of glucagon rises to twice its initial value (Esterhuizen and Howell 1970), while stimulation of the vagus nerve produced no effect. Samols, Taylor, and Kajinuma (1971, 1972) verified the stimulation of glucagon secretion by adrenaline and noradrenaline. Marliss, Girardier, Seydoux, Wollheim, Kanazawa, Orci, Renold, and Porte (1973) working with dogs have regularly been able to obtain a secretion of glucagon by the stimulation of mixed pancreatic nerves. They interpret the function of the nervous influences as an adjustment of the sensitivity of the alpha-cells to glucose. Iversen (1973) perfusing the isolated dog pancreas with physiological concentrations of adrenaline, noradrenaline and isoproterenol obtained a rise of glucagon and a drop in insulin, although with increased concentrations of glucose the glucagon should actually have fallen. The glucagon secretion with catecholamines can be neutralized by propanalol. From the researches of Iverson and according to Luyckx (1974) it can be concluded that the stimulation of glucagon secretion brought about by catecholamines is mediated by a beta-receptor and the inhibition of insulin secretion by an alpha-receptor. It should be noted that the influence of the sympathetic nervous system in encouraging glucagon secretion consequently functions through two pathways: one is neural and direct via the splanchnic nerve, while the second is indirect via the adrenal medulla and the secretion of catecholamines, which in their turn lead to the production of glucagon.

2.2.1.8. Neural Control of Insulin Secretion

Investigations concerning the physiological and pharmacological control of insulin secretion (Pfeiffer 1970, Frerichs and Creutzfeldt

	in vivo	in vitro
Glucose [a]	+	+
Mannose	+	+
Fructose	+	+
D-Ribose	+	+
D-Xylose		+
Xylitol	+	+
Ribitol		+
Leucin	+	+
Arginine	+	+
Pyruvic acid		+
β-oxybutyric [b]	+	±
Glucagon [a]	+	+
Secretin [a]	+	+
Pancreozymine	+	+
Gastrin		+
Isoprenaline [a c]	+	+
Adrenaline [d]	+	+
3′,5′-AMP [a]	±	+
Dibutyryl 3′,5′-AMP [a]	+	+
ACTH	+	+
TSH		+
STH	+	±
Sulphonylurea [a]	+	+
Insulin antibodies	+	+
Ca^{++} (necessary)		+
Theophylline	+	+
Caffeine		+
Vagus stimulation	+	

[a] Potentiated by theophyllin or caffeine.
[b] Sheep, lamb, rabbit, dog.
[c] Blocked by β-receptor blockers.
[d] In presence of α-receptor blockers.

Inhibitors of Insulin secretion (Ariens 1969)

	in vivo	in vitro
2-desoxyglucose	+	+
Manno-heptulose	+	+
Glucosamine		+
Noradrenaline [a]	+	+
Adrenaline [a]	+	+
Diazoxide	+	+
Vagotomy	+	
Insulin (high concentration)	+	+

[a] Blocked by α-receptor blockers.

Fig. 9. Releasing (upper) and inhibiting factors for insulin secretion (Ariens 1969, Pfeiffer 1969)

1971) have shown that a large number of stimulating and inhibiting, endogenous and exogenous factors is involved (Fig. 9). Further stimulating factors are glibenclamide and ethanol (ethyl alcohol) (Kuhl, Anderson *et al.* 1975) and inhibiting ones, diphenyldantoin (Malherbe 1972, Berger *et al.* 1975) cyproheptadine (Joost, Lenzen, Beckmann, and Hasselblatt 1975), thyroxine (Lenzen 1975) and somatostatin. The multifactoral regulation of insulin secretion was stressed by Malaisse (1972).

The control of insulin secretion by catecholamines and the direct neural supply of the beta-cells was first discussed by Britton (1925) after experimental hyperglycaemia and vagus stimulation. Leipert

Stimulation of adrenergic receptors	Effect on glucose-induced insulin secretion	Blocking of the adrenergic receptors
α-receptor (adrenaline, noradrenaline)	inhibition	β-receptor (Propranolol)
β-receptor (Isopropylnoradrenaline)	increase	α-receptor * (Phentolamin, phenoxy-benzamine, ergotamine)

* The inhibitory effect of adrenaline is abolished.

Fig. 10. (From Frerichs and Creutzfeldt 1971)

(1950) suspected that insulin might be the vagal hormone. Pharmacological studies on the mode of action of the catecholamines on the secretion of insulin (Senft 1967, 1968, Misbin, Edgar, and Lockwood 1970, Loubatueres 1971, Frerichs and Creutzfeldt 1971, Fussgänger, Laube, and Pfeiffer 1974) have led to the concept that the beta-cells are provided with alpha- and beta-adrenergic receptors. Noradrenaline has exclusively alpha-adrenergic actions and adrenaline has beta-adrenergic actions in addition. The net effect of the catecholamines on the beta-cells consists in the inhibition of insulin secretion mediated through the alpha-receptors. Should the beta receptors be blocked, *e.g.* by propanalol there is a more marked predominance of the catecholamine effect which is mediated through alpha-receptors, so that the inhibition of glucose-induced insulin secretion becomes still more marked. On the other hand should the alpha-receptors be inhibited, *e.g.* by phentolamine, the effect of the beta-receptors predominates and there is an increase in insulin secretion, in the same way as with stimulation of the beta-receptors by, *e.g.* isopropylnoradrenaline (Fig. 10). The pharmacological application of these blockers leads naturally, at the same time, to catecholamine-determined stimulation of glucagon secretion through alpha-receptors (Samols, Green, Tyler, and Marks 1972).

Porte, Graber, Kuzuya, and Williams (1971) and Porte (1967) have investigated the clinical significance in man of these pharmacological studies and have shown that with infusion of adrenaline the glucose-stimulated secretion of insulin does not occur, whereas this effect is prevented by previous administration of dihydro-ergotamine. Baum and Porte (1968) and Porte (1969) have pointed out the blocking of insulin secretion by operations under hypothermia which represents one of the strongest activators of the sympathetic nervous system. The inhibition of insulin secretion was reduced or prevented by rewarming and by the administration of alpha-receptors blockers. Stremmel (1974) confirmed these findings in a group of general surgical cases.

Robertson and Porte (1973) had assumed that after the use of alpha- and beta-blockers in man, that not only the glucose-stimulated, but also the basal insulin secretion was modulated by the alpha-adrenergic mechanisms. Iversen (1973) succeeded in confirming these findings in the isolated perfused dogs pancreas. Williams and Porte (1974) in their survey of the neural mechanism of insulin secretion put forward the view that adrenaline and noradrenaline are the only endogenous inhibitors of insulin secretion. Only the stimulation which is induced by arginine or secretin cannot be suppressed by catecholamines. When there is abolition of the catecholamines and their net effect on the inhibition of insulin secretion, which is mediated through the alpha receptors, we are then confronted with a hypersensitive reacting beta-cells system which shows a more intense response when stimulated. Not only the humoral catecholamines, but also the noradrenaline which is released at the sympathetic nerve ending of the beta-cells is effective here, and maintains a continuous basal influence. According to Woods and Porte there are several explanations of the almost exclusive restriction of insulin research to hormone activity. These include apparently minimal effect of pancreatic denervation on glucose metabolism, normal blood sugar values after pancreas transplantation and contradictory results in investigations on the catecholamines and in stimulation tests on the peripheral nerves.

Stimulation of the lateral nucleus of the hypothalamus leads to insulin secretion, stimulation of the ventro-medial nucleus to inhibition of insulin secretion and to a rise in glucagon. On the other hand, bilateral destruction of the ventro-medial nucleus leads to hyperphagia and to hyperinsulinism, which is primary, and is not a sequel of the hyperphagia. This concept was experimentally confirmed by Karakash, Hustvedt, le Marchand, and Jeanrenaud (1975) and Hustvedt (1975). Bajaj, Chhina, Mohankumar, Garg, and Baldev Singh (1975) have introduced stereotactic electrodes into the ventro-medial nucleus and into the lateral hypothalamus of male rhesus monkeys. After long-term tests they were able to demonstrate that after stimulation of electrodes in the ventro-lateral part of the hypothalamus there was a definite rise in insulin, and after stimulation of the ventro-medial electrodes there was a definite fall in the amount of insulin which could be measured immunologically. These authors speak of the enterohypothalamoinsulin axis. Chieri, Farina, Halparin, and Basabe (1975) after prolonged infusion of glucose into the dogs carotid artery were able to achieve a biphasic rise of insulin, which was much smaller after vagotomy and was absent after glucose infusion into the jugular vein of vagotomized dogs.

Woods and Porte allege that the smell alone and even the sight of, a splendid meal leads to insulin secretion. There is in dogs, as in man a biphasic rise of insulin after a meal. After sham feeding only the first peak appears, and giving the meal directly into the stomach leads only to the second rise, so that the initial insulin response is interpreted as purely neurogenic. Investigations in man with lemon juice and sugar were identical. Lemon juice and saccharin release the initial peak, sugar enclosed in a gelatin capsule the second. Woods and Porte conclude from the investigations, that there is always a centrally released rise in insulin, if the brain perceives a rise in glucose "relative to the periphery". Under normal conditions the basal insulin secretion is not under the control of the vagus, but the basal level is continuously monitored by the sympathetic.

For parasympathetic stimulation to be effective it is immaterial if this takes place in the lateral hypothalamic nucleus, in the motor nucleus of the vagus, on the roots of the vagus or in the mixed pancreatic nerves. Likewise the inhibition of insulin secretion and the rise in glucagon secretion can be achieved equally as well by stimulation of the ventromedial nucleus of the hypothalamus, as via the splanchnic nerves and the mixed pancreatic nerves. Findlay, Grill, Lever, Randle, and Spriggs (1969) have described a particular branch of the dorsal nucleus of the vagus, whose stimulation produced an abrupt rise of insulin. Frohman, Ezdinli, and Javid (1967) had also observed the effect of vagus stimulation on the secretion of insulin. The rise of secretion after stimulation of the dorsal vagus was also confirmed by Kaneto, Kosaka, and Nakao (1967). Orsetti and

Passebois (1975) have been able to repeat this effect on isolated pancreasvagus preparations in the rabbit, although only after blocking of the adrenergic effect and with a slightly raised blood sugar. Parasympathomimetic drugs infused into the pancreatic artery release a rise of insulin, which can be completely prevented by atropine, whereas glucose-induced insulin secretion cannot be inhibited by atropine (Kaneto, Kajinuma, Kosaka, and Nakao 1968).

Campfield and Renold succeeded in 1975 in proving the regulation even of the basal insulin secretion, by catecholamines in physiological concentrations. Concentrations of 2×10^{-9} M of noradrenaline and 10^{-10} M adrenaline acting on isolated islets cause a reproducible and dose-related fall of basal insulin secretion; this was independent of the glucose concentration. Campfield (personal communication 1975) is convinced that by direct neural stimulation, concentrations of 10^{-7} to 10^{-6} M of noradrenaline exist in the synaptic gaps and hence a far higher dose-related inhibition of insulin secretion is attained.

2.2.2. Neurohumoral Regulation

2.2.2.1. The Hypothalamic-Pituitary System

The discovery by Bargmann (1949, 1969) of "Neurokrinie", the internal secretion of hypothalamic hormones and the description of the anatomy of the hypothalamo-pituitary systems (E. Hagen 1963, Szentagothai 1965, Engelhardt 1965, Nauta and Haymaker 1969, Green 1969, and Engelhardt 1971) had led neurophysiologists and neuroendocrinologists to the concept of the hypothalamic hypophyseotropic hormones, which in their turn were released in the hypothalamus under the influence of neurotransmitters. Reports on the clinical aspects may be seen in the papers of H. Hoff (1950), Orthner (1958), F. Hoff (1965), and Scriba (1973).

The "releasing hormones" for ACTH, MSH, growth hormone, prolactin, thyrotrophin, LH and FSH have been identified, their structure has been partly identified and they have been synthesized. The inhibiting hormones for MSH, growth hormones and prolactin have been found. Also, the site of formation of the hypothalamic hormones is known to some extent—in the case of the "releasing factors" for growth hormone and ACTH it is in the ventromedial nucleus (van der Meer 1973, Krulich 1974). The hypothalamic hormones mentioned reach the hormone-producing cells of the anterior lobe through the portal vessels and stimulate or inhibit their secretion. The hormones oxytocin and vasopressin which are produced in the paraventricular and supraoptic nuclei are conducted by the axons of their neurosecretory neurones into the posterior lobe of the pituitary, where they are stored. More recent knowledge concerns the metabolic action of prolactin and of somatostatin, the GH-RIH (growth hormone release inhibiting factor) (see surveys by Scriba and Karg 1975). The latter not only inhibits the secretion of growth hormone, of gastrin and of TSH but also the pancreatic hormones insulin and glucagon in particular (Alberti *et al.* 1973). Indeed this action is independent of the presence of the pituitary, so that at the moment the therapeutic use of synthesized somatostatin, as well as other synthetic hypothalamic hormones is being discussed.

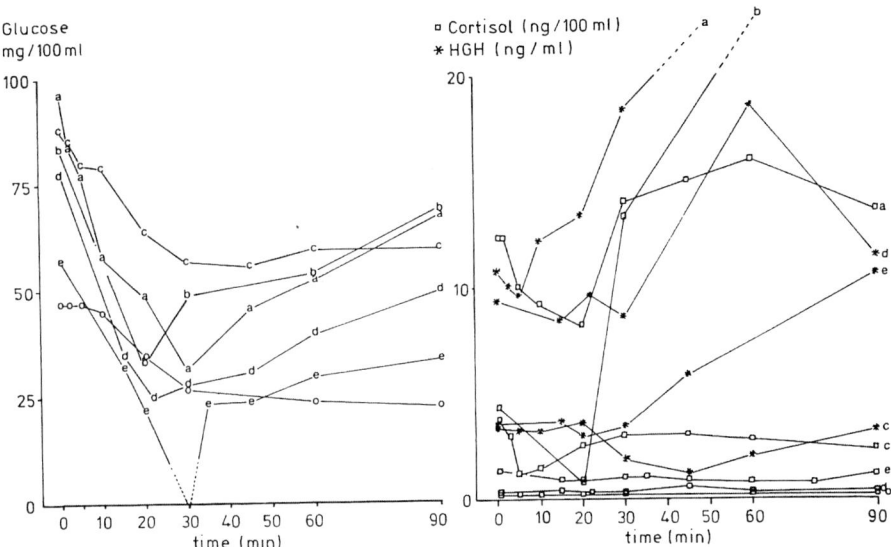

Fig. 11. *a* and *b* Normal person, rapid recovery from hypoglycaemia with a more steeply responding HGH- and cortisol-reaction. *d* Partial damage, absent rise of HGH with a normal cortisol response. *e* and *o* Very marked and sustained hypoglycaemia, with absent or minimal rise in HGH and cortisol (chromophobe adenoma, craniopharyngioma). *c* Slight hypoglycaemia with no rise of HGH and cortisol after preliminary treatment with Dexamethazone

In addition to the pituitary hormones and the hypothalamic somatostatin, which are essential for glucose metabolism, additional humoral factors in the hypothalamus have been described, which are recognized as having a direct action on carbohydrate metabolism. Carraway and Leeman (1971) have isolated from the bovine hypothalamus a polypeptide, consisting of thirteen amino-acids, which they have called neurotensin. In animal experiments this has been shown to produce cyanosis, hypotension, a rise of the LH and FSH and a marked hyperglycaemia (Carraway, Demers, and Leeman 1973). Idahl and Martin (1971) succeeded in isolating a humoral factor from the ventro-lateral hypothalamus, which stimulated the isolated islets cells to give up their insulin, while with extracts from the ventro-medial hypothalamus no such effects can be detected (Martin et al. 1973).

The "neuroendocrine integration" (E. Scharrer 1966) and the "governing principles of the adeno-hypophyseal internal secretion" (Weissbecker 1965) require anatomically intact and functioning structures in the hypothalamus, and in the pituitary and its stalk. The circadian rhythm of the secretion of cortisol or ACTH and growth hormone (Krieger 1971, Vasquez 1973) and the negative feedback system between cortisol and the ACTH releasing factor are disturbed by structural lesions. Insulin-induced hypoglycaemia is marked and sustained, if the pituitary stalk is divided or if active pituitary tissue is absent (Fig. 11). The increased sensitivity to insulin of hypo-physectomized patients (Oberdisse 1953, Oberdisse and Tönnis 1953) and in patients with pituitary tumours (Marguth 1964) has been established. With them and with most patients with craniopharyngi-oma there is no possibility of a neurohumoral reaction to hypo-glycaemia, with ACTH (i.e. cortisol) and growth hormone.

2.2.2.2. Glucose-Sensitive Neurones in the Hypothalamus

Numerous stimuli such as every type of physical and psychical pain, stress, severe bodily exertion, drugs, amino-acids and hypoglycaemia are able to encourage the secretion of these hormones which are important for the regulation of the carbohydrate metabo-lism, while the rhythm of sleep and waking influences the circadian secretion. On the other hand glucose is able to lower the level of growth hormone and cortisol immediately. This reaction and the secretion of ACTH and cortisol in response to glucopaenia indicate that the level of the blood sugar is controlled in the region of the hypothalamus in the same way as osmolarity and the core tem-perature, and also that a control mechanism which has hormonal and neural effectors as described also exists for glucose.

In fact, Oomura et al. (1964, 1969) by systematic administration of glucose and by electro-osmotic application of glucose by means of a micropipette have been successful in changing the activity of a great number of individual neurones in the hypothalamus (Fig. 12). A half of the neurones in the ventro-medial nucleus which were tested reacted to a rise of glucose with an increase of the neuronal discharges per unit of time, the remainder showed no change; in the lateral hypothalamus a third of the neurones tested responded to a rise of glucose, a quarter however were susceptible to a lowering of the glucose concentration and the remainder showed no change.

A large number of neurones were investigated in the cerebral cortex, in the thalamus and in other structures without any glucose sensitive cells being found.

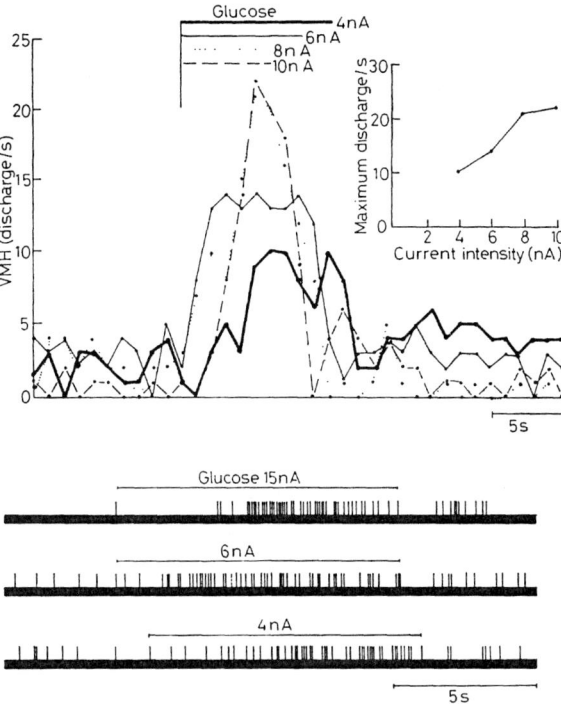

Fig. 12. *Upper:* Dose-related changes in the discharge frequency of a neurone from the ventro-medial nucleus of the hypothalamus, before, during, and after electro-osmotic application of glucose. *Lower:* Modulation of neuronal activity of another cell from the ventro-medial hypothalamus by glucose. This cell also increased its discharge rate in relation to the dose. None of the glucose sensitive cells reacted to the administration of sodium. (After Oomura *et al.* 1969)

These findings support the hypothesis of a monitoring device for the glucose level, situated in the hypothalamus, which has an unequal number of plus and minus sensors. The schematic "glucostat" according to Schade (Fig. 13) shows a finer division of the scale for increases in the glucose, and the "set point" is immediately adjustable by means of the neural input.

Long-term changes as a result of hypothalamic lesions lead to a loss of glucose sensors and hence to aphagia or hyperphagia. Bilateral destruction of the ventro-medial nuclei leads to excessive obesity, but a bilateral lesion of the lateral hypothalamus is only followed by an extreme emaciation, if parts of the ventromedial nucleus are pre-served. Thus, it is very rarely met with in the clinical material.

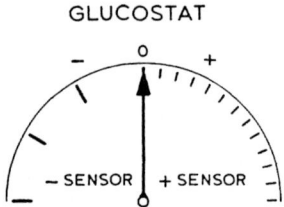

Fig. 13. Schematic representation of the glucostat. Note the difference in scale for the negative and positive part of the sensing device. (After Schade 1970)

2.2.2.3. Effect of the Location of Diencephalic Lesions on the Clinical and Endocrine Symptoms

In clinical research the influence of cerebral and intracranial diseases on the endocrine system is very difficult to demarcate. On the one hand a slowly-growing tumour with extensive neurological deficits will only displace the hypothalamo-pituitary system, but leave it functionally intact, whereas on the other hand very small acute lesions can lead to complete failure of the endocrine regulation but, at the same time elude clinical, neurological or radiological detection.

Histories recorded in a group of neurosurgical material include an ependymal cyst of the third ventricle with insulin-resistant diabetes mellitus (Byrow and Russell 1932), a midbrain cyst with insulin-refractory hyperglycaemia (Penfield 1934), a ventro-medial tumour with obesity and post-operatively a secondary uncontrollable hyper-glycaemia (Reeves and Plum 1969), chronic effects on water metabo-lism and energy balance, disturbances of temperature regulation, of sleep and of behaviour and a hyperglycaemia resistant to treatment after a second operation on a craniopharyngioma (Killeffer and Stern 1970). It is common to the cases described that the hyperglycaemia does not represent an isolated symptom but is only one single aspect of an extensive disturbance of regulation in the endocrine system. Oppenheimer (1967) described four personal cases with pan-hypo-pituitarism and galactorrhoea in sarcoidosis of the central nervous system, pinealoma and a suprasellar craniopharyngioma and also a meningioma in the region of the chiasm. Reference is made to the difficulty in interpreting the endocrinological findings in relation to the location of central lesions. In 1959 Bauer reviewed sixty cases of hypothalamic diseases and reported that the most frequent symptom is a failure of sexual development or sexual function, and this mostly with lesions in the anterior and inferior parts of the hypothalamus, while a pubertus praecox appeared frequently with lesions in the posterior hypothalamus and in the mamillary bodies (Spatz 1955). Damage to the hypothalamus which weighs a mere four grams and is 2.5 cm long, leads to syndromes of stimulation and deficits and not to specific symptoms.

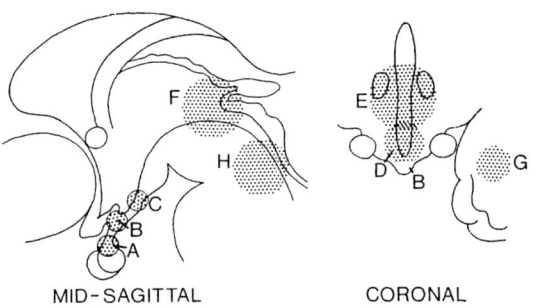

MID-SAGITTAL   CORONAL

Fig. 14. (After Rothballer 1966)

Wild and Simon (1950) and Oberdisse (1951) have investigated the relationship between organic lesions in the region of the hypothalamus and pituitary and carbohydrate metabolism, and by using insulin stress they were not able to draw any conclusions regarding the location of the lesion. Rothballer (1966) in his survey of the endocrine manifestations of central nervous diseases stressed that the site was a decisive factor in the endocrine picture. Total suprasellar lesions with damage to the infundibulum and stalk leads to a non-reacting system working on the basal hormone level, in which there is only an excessive secretion of prolactin. The response to stress, hyper- and hypoglycaemia fails, as also does the circadian cortisol rhythm. Low section or damage (A) (Fig. 14) to the stalk leads to division of the portal vessels and hence to extensive infarction of the anterior pituitary. The appearance of diabetes insipidus is only transitory, as the neurosecretory pathways are preserved and their hormones can be discharged into the general circulation via the stalk. The isolated high lesion (B) is rare; the adenohypophysis produces a basal hormone level, which however can be stimulated by the exogenous "releasing" hormone. In this instance the diabetes insipidus is permanent.

Para-infundibular lesions (C) leave intact the effector, the hypo-thalamo-pituitary tract; however homeostasis is disturbed as the corresponding sensor or the "set point" is damaged and the control mechanism thereby suffers an unregulated overaction. Lesions in the region such as hamartoma, ectopic pinealoma, ependymoma, tuberose sclerosis and even hydrocephalus of the third ventricle can lead to pubertus praecox (Spatz 1955). Partial lesions, principally a deficit of the gonadotropins, can arise through slowly-growing infundibular lesions (D), which together with the well-known obesity of the ventromedial lesions, constitutes the classic Fröhlich's syndrome. All these lesions can be associated with disturbances of emotion, consciousness and energy metabolism. Periventricular and dorsally situated bilateral lesions (E) show emotional, consciousness and temperature disturbances and also epileptic attacks and autonomic phenomena (Penfield 1934), without anything of note being apparent in the endocrine system. With extrahypothalamic lesions (F, G, H) clearly circumscribed endocrine manifestations have not been described, abnormalities of the corticoid rhythm are known in quadrigeminal and temporal lobe lesions. In lesions of the upper brain stem with disturbances of consciousness the daily rhythm is abolished.

2.3. Summary

In the hypothalamus is the region, where afferents arrive via neural pathways and the blood level, and by means of a monitoring mechanism for glucose, efferent mechanisms for influencing the glucose metabolism are initiated. These operate firstly in the central nervous neural control of the internal organs, and secondly in the regulation of the secretion of the pituitary hormones.

The neural connexion between hypothalamus and liver cells facilitates the direct control of the activity of key enzymes of glycogenolysis and glycogen synthesis. The immediate neural inhibition of insulin secretion and the encouragement of glucagon secretion in the pancreas and the swift stimulation of the adrenal medulla represent a rapid and efficient mechanism against the danger of hypoglycaemia and on the other hand contribute to the urgent supply of energy.

The neural influences are supplemented by the secretion of pituitary hormones, in particular by ACTH and hence glucocorticoids and growth hormone, which like the neural mechanisms are controlled by the hypothalamus. The hormonal action on the glucose metabolism which is partly delayed, takes place after some hours, its more acute effect is still being discussed to some extent. Through the discovery of somatostatin and its inhibitory effect on growth hormone, insulin and glucagon, another effective mechanism of the hypothalamus has come to light (Sieradski, Schatz, Nierle, and Pfeiffer 1975, and Garcia and Rosselin 1975). A concentration of 1 ng/ml leads to maximal inhibition of glucagon- and insulin-secretion (Iversen 1975) even if their secretion is being stimulated by other factors such as glucose, tolbutamide, arginine or catecholamines. It will be the aim of future investigations to determine if such concentrations of somatostatin appear physiologically in man and hence whether any corresponding effects of the hypothalamus on the pancreatic hormones are possible.

3. Methods Employed

3.1. Standardization of the Withdrawal of Blood

All blood samples were venous. Fasting values and tolerance loads were estimated between 8.0 and 10.0 a.m. and in every case were undertaken after 12 hours abstinence from any oral and intravenous food intake. If a full normal diet were not possible, the feeding of the patients was achieved in a standardized manner with intravenous and tube feeding with a total intake of circa 2,400 calories, which was divided between carbohydrates, fat and protein in the proportion 60 : 20 : 20.

3.2. Standardization of the Loading Tests

3.2.1. Intravenous Glucose Load

After determination of the fasting values, 0.33 g glucose/kg body weight were given intravenously over a period of two minutes. The first specimen was taken after two minutes and the following after ten, fourteen, eighteen, twenty-two and sixty-minutes. In particular cases specimens were taken at additional times. The urine produced during this time was collected in order to estimate the amount of sugar excreted. The blood sugar level was estimated immediately after the end of the "stress" test. For the hormone analyses the sera were frozen and dealt with in larger series. The specimens for glucagon estimation were collected in previously cooled plastic tubes and mixed with a drop of heparin and circa 1,000 units of Trasolyl to 10 ml of blood, and only subsequently centrifuged and frozen. The intravenous glucose lead ("stress") was done pre-operatively and repeated on the first and seventh post-operative days, after cranio-cerebral injuries it was done on the first and seventh day. The physiological oral glucose tolerance test was not undertaken, in favour of the intravenous, as numerous inponderables influence the oral absorption of the glucose in the post-operative phase.

3.2.2. Insulin Hypoglycaemia

0.1 i.u./kg body weight of old insulin intravenously. Blood is taken at the start and ofter 10, 15, 20, 25, 30, 35, 45, 60 and 90 minutes.

3.2.3. Arginine "Stress"

Arginine monohydrochloride infusion is given within a half hour, in a dose of 30 g in adults and 0.5 g/kg body weight in children. Blood taken at 0, 15, 30, 40, 60, 90 and 120 minutes.

3.2.4. Somatostatin Load

After withdrawal of the fasting sample 250 pg of somatostatin were given intravenously as a bolus and 750 pg as a following drip infusion through the next 60 minutes. Specimens were taken at 15, 30, 45 and 60 minutes, sometimes after 90 and 120 minutes in addition.

3.3. Chemical Estimation Methods

3.3.1. Glucose

The blood sugar level was estimated with the aid of a semi-automatic glucose analyser made by Beckman and Co. The estimation of D-glucose took place by the GOD method, according the Bernt and Lachenicht (1974).

3.3.2. Free Fatty Acids

The estimation of free fatty acids which was undertaken in certain cases was modelled on the method of Duncombe (1964) and was performed with a commercially available reagent kit.

3.3.3. Human Growth Hormone (HGH)

The radioimmunoassay of growth hormone of Sorin and Co., Italy, was used for growth hormone (Molinatti, Massara, Strumia, Pennise, Scassellatti, Vancheri 1969, Nieschlag, Wombacher, Kroeger, and Oversier 1971). This uses a second antibody for the separation of the marked hormone bound to the first antibody. The total complex formed in this way is centrifuged several times and the supernatant drawn off, so that the residual activity can be measured in a gamma-counter (Biogamma, Beckman and Co.). The specivity of the antiserum and the higher degree of purity of the growth hormone preparation was established by Molinatti *et al.* The test of sensitivity, as the lowest concentration

significantly distinguishable from 0 yielded a value of 0.1 ng/ml. All
the values of the standard curve and also each specimen of the serum
to be estimated, were assessed three times.

In co-operation with the mathematicians Oscar Hoffman and
W. Muller the evaluation of the date was mechanized with the help
of an electronic date processor, employing the Spline approximation
(Marscher, Dobby, Erhardt, Landersdorf, Popp, Ringel, and Scriba
1974, Marschner, Erhardt, and Scriba 1974) (Fig. 15).

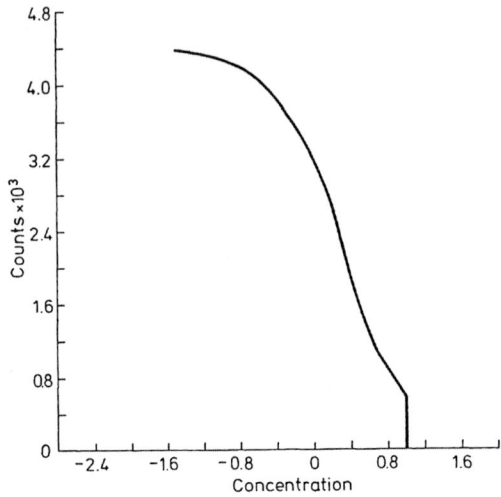

Fig. 15. Original standard curve for HGH using the Spline approximation

3.3.4. Insulin

The estimation of insulin was performed with the kit sold by
Pharmacia Limited. In contrast to the double antibody method, the
antibodies here are bound to Sephadex particles, so that the separation of the bound from the free action of radio-activity by means of
centrifuging is simple and less time-consuming. Here also each estimation of the standard values and of the specimens was carried out three
times.

3.3.5. Cortisol

The estimation of cortisol in plasma was performed by K. Hacken-
berg (Endocrinological Department of the First Medical Clinic of
the Ruhr University in Essen) using the competitive protein-binding
method (B. P. Murphy, W. Engerburg, and C. J. Pattee 1963,
B. P. Murphy 1967, 1969).

3.3.6. Glucagon

The radioimmunoassay of glucagon was undertaken by E. Samols (Louisville, Kentucky, U.S.A.). The pancreas specific glucagon antiserum 30 K prepared by R. Unger (Dallas, Texas) was used.

3.3.7. Catecholamines

The urinary catecholamines were estimated in the Biochemical Institute of the University of Giessen by the modified method of Staudinger.

3.4. Pharmacokinetics of Glucose

Since the fundamental researches of Conard (1955) the so-called K-value has been used as the standard for the assessment of glucose utilization. Here, it refers to a constant, which on a semi-logarithmic grid describes the slope of the straight line, which results from the fall in concentration of glucose after a standardized intravenous glucose "load". The constant is a function of the quotient from ln 2 and the "half-life" period of the substance which can be read off the straight line (Fig. 16).

In the foregoing studies the utilization of glucose was investigated according to pharmacokinetic principles (Dost 1968, Dost, Gladtke, v. Hattingberg, and Ring 1968, v. Hattingberg, Gladtke, and Dost 1970, Gladtke and v. Hattingberg 1973, v. Hattingberg 1973, v. Hattingberg, Dost, and Gladtke 1973).

After a disturbance of the steady state by an intravenous loading the organism endeavours by elimination, by metabolizing and excretion, to restore the original equilibrium. After the distribution in the body compartments the fall of concentration in the blood follows an exponential pattern in that the blood level falls in proportion to the concentration from time to time. On a semi-logarithmic grid this curve turns out as a straight line (Fig. 17).

According to Dost and v. Hattingberg and in contrast to Conard the blood sugar concentration is obtained after deduction of the fasting value, which is regarded as zero value.

Gladtke and v. Hattingberg (1973) have shown that it is only after deduction of the zero (fasting) value that the exponential function, and hence the straight line, results (Fig. 18). With glucose and with substances foreign to the body its was shown that the elimination half-life value is a constant if the "zero" value is taken into consideration in absent (nil), low and raised fasting values (Fig. 19).

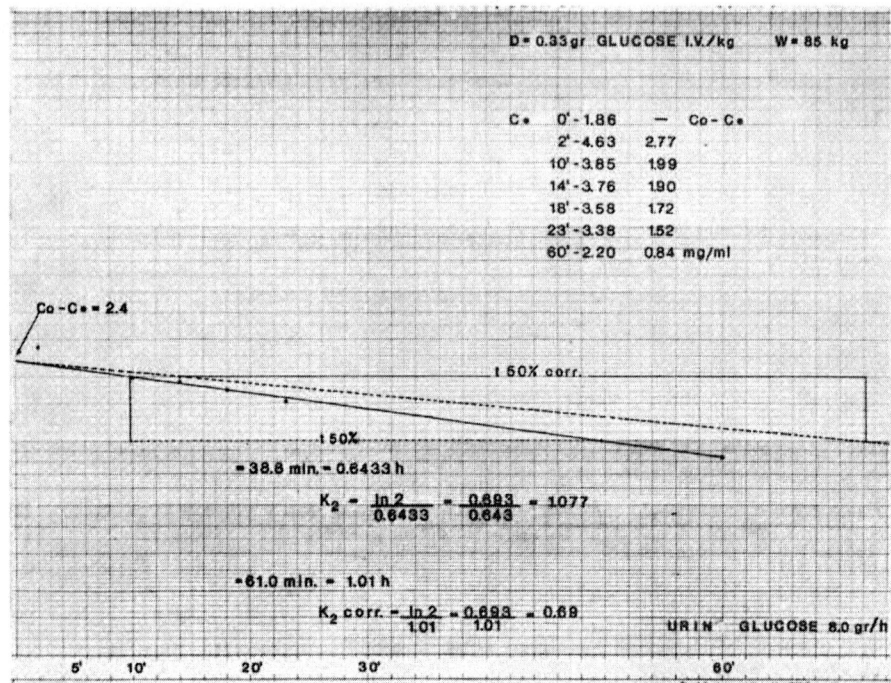

Fig. 16. (See text)

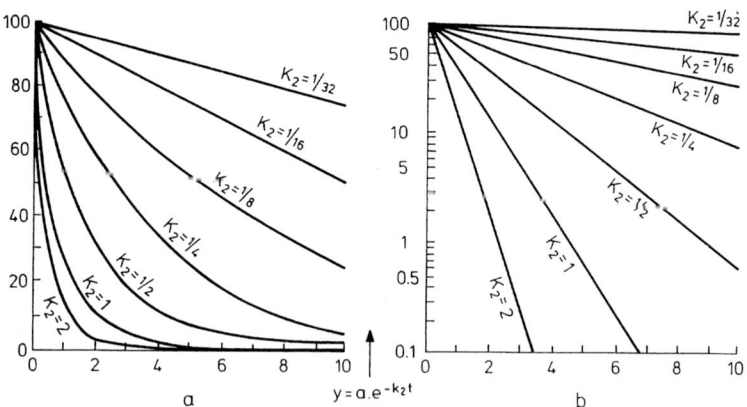

Fig. 17. Groups of curves on a linear (a) and a semi-logarithmic (b) grid. The slope of the respective lines indicates the elimination constant k_2. (After Gladtke and v. Hattingberg 1973)

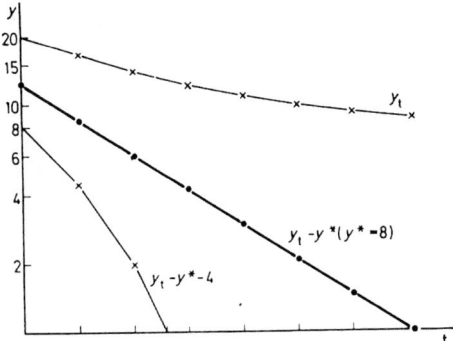

Fig. 18. Exponential function on a semi-logarithmic grid $(y_t - y^*)$. Concentration-curve without deduction of the fasting value (y_t), concentration-curve after deduction of a too large fasting value $(y_t - y^* - 4)$

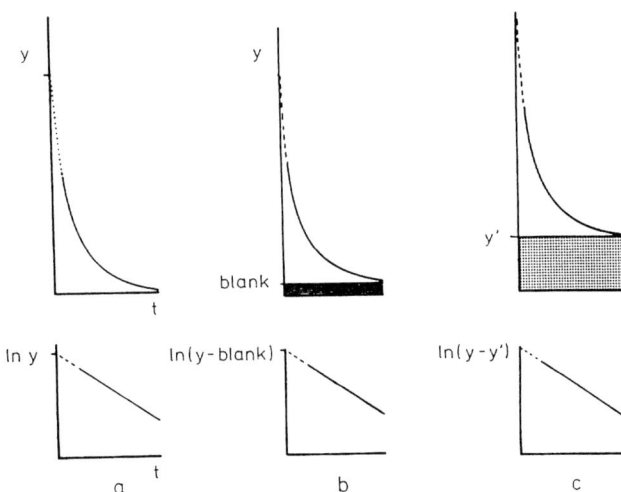

Fig. 19. a) Intravenous load, b) with the "zero" value (blank), c) with fasting value in the test subjects (y^*). (After Gladtke and v. Hattingberg 1973)

The pharmacokinetic analysis of the pattern of concentrations furnishes further data which can be used in assessing the situation in the metabolism of glucose. By extrapolation of the straight line as far as the zero time, the estimated initial concentration can be obtained, which would be present, if a diffusion balance could be obtained immediately at the moment of injection. From this estimated initial concentration one is able to calculate the partition volumes or the distribution constant:

$V = D : y\,O$ (D = dose, $y\,O$ = estimated initial concentration) or if related to the body weight (kg):

$\Delta' = D/kg : y\,O$.

The multiplication of the partition volume of a substance by the fasting value yields the total amount contained therein ($y^* \times V$, or corrected to the body weight $y^* \times \Delta'$).

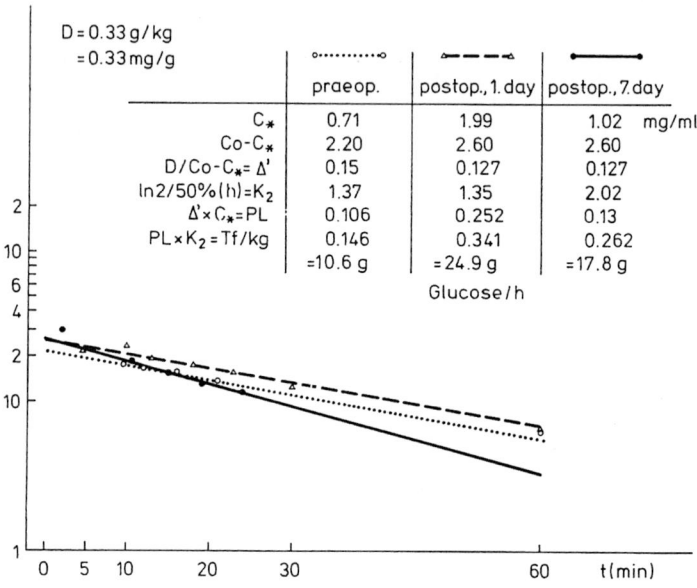

Fig. 20. An example of pharmacokinetic data pre-operatively and on the first and seventh post-operative days. *D* dose, *C* fasting value, *Co-C** estimated initial concentration, Δ' distribution coefficient, K_2 elimination constant, *PL* pool, *Tf* turnover (transfer)

The amount of glucose is called the easily available glucose pool (Fig. 20).

The constant designated as "rate constant of elimination" K 2 indicates how often the amount contained in the pool is exchanged or eliminated in a unit of time. According to Dost by multiplying the pool with K 2 the "transfer" or turnover (Tf) is calculated. This procedure is of practical value for our investigations, in that, by mathematical analysis of the course of the concentrations evidence can be obtained regarding the absolute amount of glucose transferred per unit of time. In addition, the half-life concept introduced by Dost has the advantage that it provides data which allow a direct comparison in different persons regardless of their size, surface area and weight.

For plotting (straight line) on the semi-logarithmic grid four to five blood samples were used in the period from 10–22 minutes after a standardized intravenous glucose load, with 0.33 g per kg/body weight. We did not take into consideration measurements before the tenth minute, as up to this time the distribution was still taking place, or those after the 22nd minute on account of the complex counter-regulation which was coming into action. All curves were plotted by hand, and the elimination half-life and the estimated initial concentration read off. If as a result of the glucose "load" there was excretion of glucose in the urine, the amount given intravenously was mathematically corrected according to the pharmakokinetic data using the method of v. Hattingberg.

3.5. Statistical Methods

The extensive data were collected on punch cards, stored on magnetic tape and processed with the CS 3300 at the University Computer Centre of the Justus Liebig University Giessen.

Mean (values) were calculated by the formula

$$\bar{x} = \frac{1}{n} \sum_1^n x_i$$

and the standard deviation by

$$s = \sqrt{\frac{\sum_1^n (x_i - \bar{x})^2}{n-1}}$$

For each of the means thus obtained the tolerance of the confidence interval (error of the mean) were calculated by

$$F = t_p (n-1) \cdot \frac{s}{\sqrt{n}}$$

(Kreysig 1969, Sachs 1969, Pfanzagel 1966).

With a mean calculation in relation to the frequency distributions a significant level of $p = 0.95$ was chosen, in all other instances one of $p = 0.90$ particularly for the estimation of the curves for the error of the mean.

For the statistical comparison of two groups, as well as for the correlation tests we chose distribution free methods.

The Wilcoxon test was used for tests on differing means of figures in two groups (Pfanzagel and Sachs) in which the significance of $p = 0.05$ was taken as a basis.

Correlation analysis was obtained by Spearman's coefficient of rank correlation (Pfanzagel) with a significance level of $p = 0.05$.

Calculation of mean concentrations:

The average changing values between the times t_a and t_e (here the concentration in question) were obtained from

$$M = \frac{1}{t_e - t_a} \int_{t_a}^{t_e} y(t)\, dt$$

if the changing course of the averaged values is designated as $y(t)$.

As the continually changing value of the function $y(t)$ is not known, because the concentrations $y(t_i) = y_i$ $(i = 1 \cdot n)$ were only measured at discret times t_i $(i = 1 \cdot n)$, the integral $1 \cdot n$ (or $1 \times n$) is approximately calculated using the trapezoidal rule (Willers 1957, Nitsche 1968) and in this way the mean value of the figure $y(t)$ over the period t_a to t_e is obtained.

$$M = \frac{1}{t_e - t_a} \sum_{1}^{n-1} \frac{y_i + y_{i+1}}{2} \cdot (t_{i+1} - t_i)$$

$(t_1 = t_a, t_n = t_e)$.

4. Results

4.1. Survey of Material and Subdivision into Groups

The investigations presented here on the regulation of glucose metabolism were undertaken in the years 1972 to 1975 on a total of 207 people. Among these were 158 test subjects on whom 240 glucose tolerance tests were performed. In 49 patients the spontaneous pattern as well as arginine and insulin stress were investigated.

The subdivision into twelve groups was done according to clinical neurological and radiological criteria taking into consideration the main site of the injury and the level of the lesion. The formation of subgroups resulted from the necessary consideration of the time of the injury for the assessment of glucose metabolism.

Group 1 (control group):

This consisted of healthy volunteers (members of the clinic, students, etc.) without regard to age, sex and normal (or ideal) weight. Any selection according to these factors was not undertaken. As the variation in glucose tolerance and insulin secretion determined by these factors (Beaser 1967, Carroll and Nestel 1973) applied in the same way to the patients in the other groups, they were also investigated as an unselected group (n = 22).

Group 2:

This included patients with obvious diabetes mellitus without any central nervous disorder (fasting hyperglycaemia, glycosuria, treatment with diet and oral antidiabetics and/or insulin) (n = 9).

Group 3 a:

This included all intracranial space-occupying lesions without regard to duration, history, location (site) and type diagnosis. The common characteristic is the pre-operative state, with no loss or impairment of consciousness (n = 68) (endocrine inactive intra- and supra-sellar pituitary tumours 29, endocrine active eosinophil adenoma 14, para-hypothalamic tumours 16, cerebral hemisphere tumours in the vicinity of the cortex 9).

Group 3 b:

The follow up of these patients on the first post-operative day is summarized here (47). In addition traumatic brain lesions (12) about one day after the injury are included here (n = 59).

Group 3 c:

Follow-up investigations of these patients on the 7th post-operative day are given here (n = 31).

Group 4 a:

In this group are included all intrasellar and suprasellar endocrine inactive pituitary tumours. Having regard to the clinical and radiological findings, the size and direction of growth of the tumour and the findings at operation, it is assumed that in these tumours there is no evidence of hypothalamic disturbance (n = 29).

Group 4 b:

Follow-up investigations of these patients on the first post-operative day (n = 17).

Group 4 c:

Further examination of these patients on the 7th post-operative day (n = 10).

Group 5 a:

This includes patients with clinical acromegaly, with radiological, operative and biopsy evidence of a pituitary tumour and endocrinological evidence of a pathological HGH secretion (n = 14).

Group 5 b:

Follow-up of these patients on the first post-operative day (n = 7).

Group 5 c:

Includes those followed up on the 7th post-operative day (n = 9).

Group 6:

Here we collected those patients from Groups 1 and 7 in whom one could assume clinical and endocrinological evidence of anterior pituitary insufficiency (basal cortisol, failure of circadian rhythm, failure of gonadotropins, hypothyroid metabolic state, absent or only basic level of HGH, HGH secretion not stimulated by hypoglycaemia and arginine) (n = 16).

Group 7 a:

This consisted of patients with space-occupying intracranial lesions in whom there was clinical, radiological and biopsy evidence of mechanical changes, chronic injury and displacement of the hypothalamus (n = 16) (bilateral olfactory groove meningioma 3, cranio-pharyngioma 3, tuberculum sellae meningioma 2, spongioblastoma of the third ventricle 2, astrocytoma of the diencephalon, optic nerve glioma, fronto-basal teratoma, malformation tumour (hamartoma) of pituitary stalk, suprasellar adenoma 2).

Group 7 b:
Follow-up of these patients on the first post-operative day (n = 13).

Group 8 a:
Patients with superficial cortical cerebral hemisphere tumours without impairment of consciousness (n = 9).

Group 8 c:
Follow-up of these patients on the first post-operative day (n = 9).

Group 8 c:
Further examination of these patients on the 7th post-operative day (n = 5).

Group 9:
Unconscious patients with the clinical signs of an acute mid-brain decerebration (mid-brain syndrome) from various causes, were in-cluded here. In these, on the basis of the clinical findings, we assumed a "transverse brain-stem injury" (Lausberg 1970), below the red nucleus and above the vestibular nucleus (Pia 1957). This clear-cut clinical syndrome is characterized by unconsciousness, extensor spasms or synergies appearing either spontaneously or on sensory stimuli, bilateral extensor plantar responses, and also by hyperventilation, hyperthermia, a rise in blood pressure and pulse rate. The patients were investigated about 24 hours after the appearance of these symp-toms, unless otherwise specified (n = 13).

Group 10:
This comprises unconscious patients with the clinical symptoms of a lesion of the pons and medulla, actually more than a midbrain syndrome (mesencephalo-ponto-bulbar lesion). The site of the func-tional, or even anatomical, brain stem lesion is considered to be at the level of the vestibular nucleus or caudal to that (Pia 1957, 1973). The clinical state is recognized by cerebral coma, reduction of tone in the muscles of the extremities, loss of muscle stretch reflexes, loss of corneal reflexes and pupillary reaction (bilateral dilated and inactive pupils), by normo- or hypothermia, absence of the vestibulo-ocular reflexes and central disturbances of respiration of various types (Pia

1957, Seeger 1968, Lausberg 1972). These investigations were also carried out a few hours up to 24 hours after the appearance of symptoms (n = 8).

Group 11:

The common characteristic of this group is the presence of cerebral coma without considering the cause, the site or level of the lesion. The patients cannot be roused, even by severe painful stimuli. They are taken from Groups 3 b, 7 b, 9 and 10 (n = 29).

Group 12:

Into this group were put unconscious patients with clinical signs of central death from known cerebral causes. The criteria for the diagnosis of brain death were: areflexia, no reactions, deep coma with no response to any stimuli, failure of respiration and temperature regulation, widely dilated inactive pupils, flaccid muscle tone and absence of extrinsic and intrinsic reflexes, isoelectric EEG (Lorenz 1969). In a few cases also evidence of brain death was shown angiographically by the arrest of the cerebral circulation. The investigation was done at varying times after the onset of brain death and hence at varying body temperatures (n = 9).

4.2. Preliminary Studies

Whilst carrying out clinical investigations on central dysregulation of autonomic functions, disturbances of metabolism, of water, electrolytes and energy metabolism were observed (Wesemann and Grote 1971). Patients with brain tumours and acute traumatic injuries to the hypothalamus showed, apart from a diabetes insipidus, a rising hyperglycaemia going from normal levels up to an uncontrollable figure of 2,000 mg%. High doses of insulin (300 i.u./day, and more) could not prevent this rise. The close relationship of this metabolic breakdown with the acute cerebral lesion was obvious, both as regards time and aetiology. We lost all patients who showed this pattern. Preliminary investigations (1970) showed that patients with the signs of dysregulation of autonomic function who survived (n = 159), only occasionally showed elevation of the blood sugar over 200 mg%. On the other hand, in patients with central dysregulation who failed to survive, a spontaneous hyperglycaemia over 200 mg% was found in 75%.

Since 1971, systematic and purposeful investigations of the central nervous disturbance of glucose metabolism were undertaken.

4.3. Spontaneous Behaviour

The disturbance of blood sugar homeostasis which appears in acute cerebral disorders, injuries and complications, may be illustrated by a few examples of the spontaneous course of events.

4.3.1. Severe Closed Craniocerebral Injury, Acute Subdural Haematoma, Secondary Coma and Midbrain Syndrome

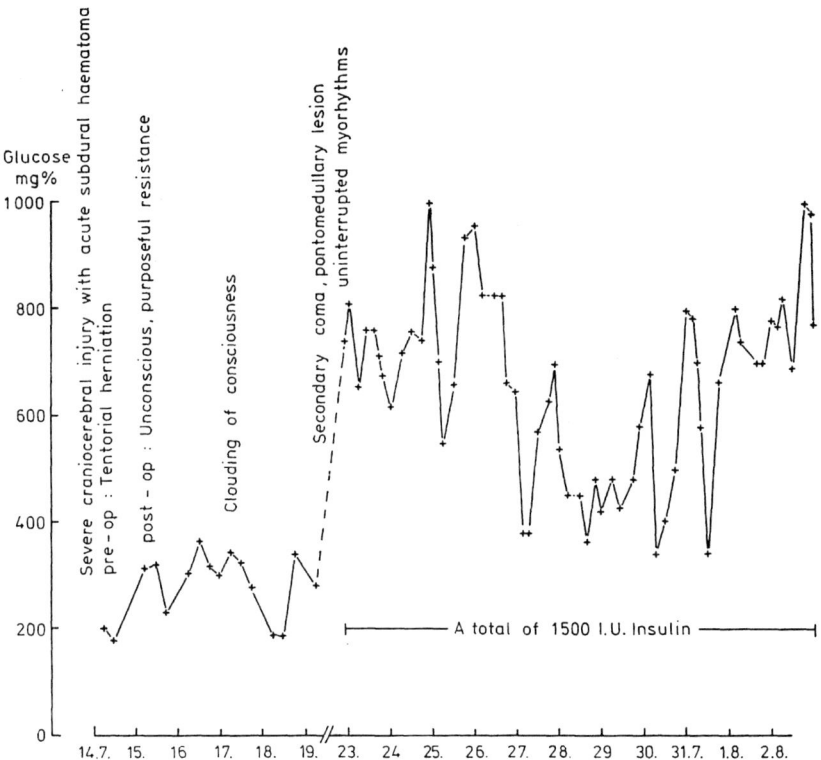

Fig. 21. Blood sugar values in a 25-year-old man (Fig. 21) after severe closed cranio-cerebral injury with standard intravenous and tube feeding. After operation on an acute haematoma the mid-brain syndrome present pre-operatively is no longer apparent. In succeeding days the injured man remained stuporose, but with increasingly prompt reactions. The blood sugar fluctuated between 180 and 350 mg%. On the 10th day secondary coma and a mid-brain syndrome which progressed by the 15th day to a mesencephalo-ponto-bulbar lesion. The spontaneous blood sugar values climbed to values of 600 to 900 mg% and are not obviously affected by giving insulin. For a few days the blood sugar fluctuated between 400 and 600 mg% and some days before his death from circulatory and renal failure, with persistent cerebral coma, the values were between 700 and 800 mg%

4.3.2. Acute Midbrain Syndrome with Extensive Intracranial Haemorrhage

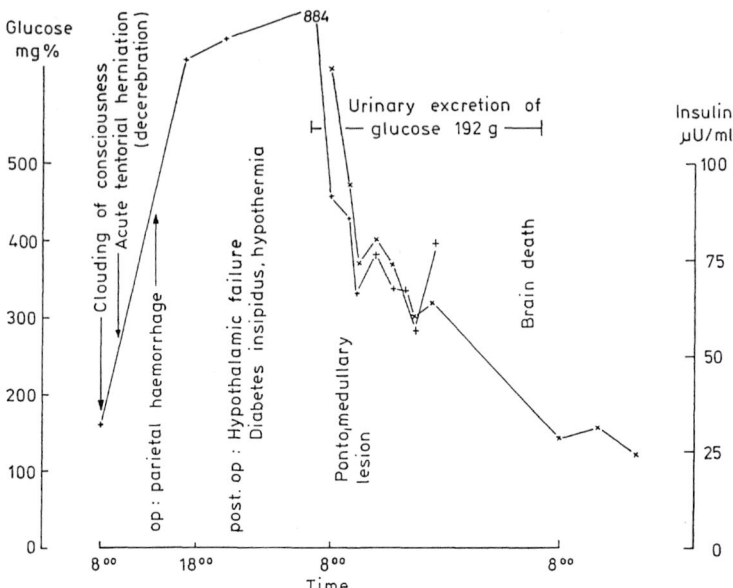

Fig. 22. A 30-year-old man without any previous history, who in a matter of days developed clouding of consciousness and signs of a hemisphere lesion. The blood sugar was 160 mg%. He developed acutely a mid-brain (tentorial) herniation, which was caused by a massive parietal haemorrhage. After confirmation the haematoma was removed. Post-operatively, with hypothermia, he developed an excessive urinary output and clinical signs of an incomplete bulbar syndrome. Spontaneous blood sugar values were between 600 and 900 mg%. Within ten hours, during the transition to a bulbar syndrome, the blood sugar fell spontaneously to 300–400 mg%. The endogenous Insulin concentrations remained high and ran parallel to the changes in the blood sugar. With the onset of brain death the blood sugar fell to normal values. Within 24 hours 192 g of glucose were excreted in the urine. At autopsy a cortical venous thrombosis was found as the cause of the mass haemorrhage. Numerous fresh spherical haemorrhages could be seen in the pons and midbrain as a result of the tentorial herniation

4.3.3. Severe Craniocerebral Injury, Acute Hypothalamic Damage

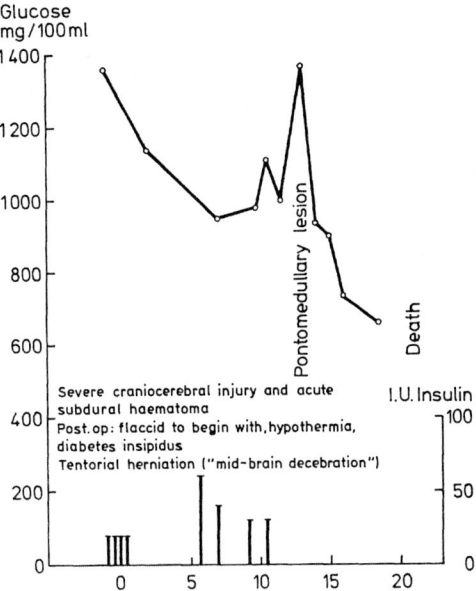

Fig. 23. A ten-year-old girl with severe craniocerebral injury and acute subdural haemorrhage. Pre-operatively an incomplete bulbar syndrome, post-operatively in addition marked hypothermia (32° rectal) and diabetes insipidus. Hours later the clinical symptoms of midbrain decerebration appeared. At this stage the spontaneous blood sugar was around 1,000 mg% and after a few hours, in spite of giving insulin it rose still higher. After some further hours the clinical signs of brain death appeared

4.3.4. Acute Hypothalamic Damage with Transition into a Midbrain Syndrome, Bulbar Damage and Brain Death After Embolization of an A.V. Angioma

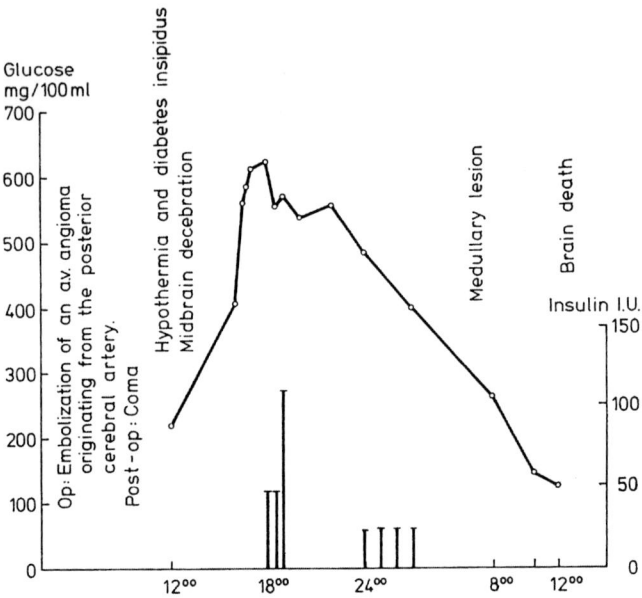

Fig. 24. This involved a 37-year-old man without any previous non-neurological history. As a complication after embolization of an AV angioma arising from the posterior cerebral artery, he suffered from occlusion of the vessels of the brain stem. Post-operatively he developed a cerebral coma and the blood sugar rose to 225 g%. After this, hypothermia and diabetes insipidus appeared and a few hours later the clinical signs of midbrain syndrome in addition. The blood sugar rose uncontrollably to 500 to 600 mg% and high doses of insulin would not bring it down. Twenty-four hours later he reached the state of bulbar damage and brain death, at which time the blood sugar was within normal limits

4.3.5. Hypothalamic Damage After Operation on a Medial
Sphenoidal Wing Meningioma

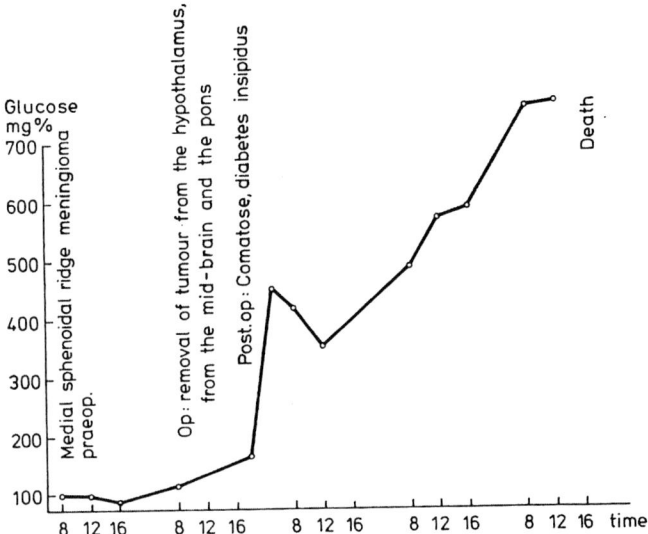

Fig. 25. In a 54-year-old man with a medially-placed sphenoidal wing meningioma, the pre-operative blood sugar was normal. At the operation the tumour was freed from the hypothalamus, mid-brain and pons. Post-operatively the patient was comatose. This state developed before the appearance of the elevated blood sugar and subsequently an uncontrollable hyperglycaemia appeared: on painful stimuli there was a tendency to extension movements in all four extremities and death occurred with clinical signs of lung oedema

4.4. Intravenous "Stress" (Load)
with Glucose 0.33 g/kg Body Weight

The original curves as plotted by the computer were taken over unchanged. The portrayal of the results of the intravenous glucose load in the various groups was obtained from the mean and the confidence interval.

4.4.1. Healthy Subjects

Individual Examples

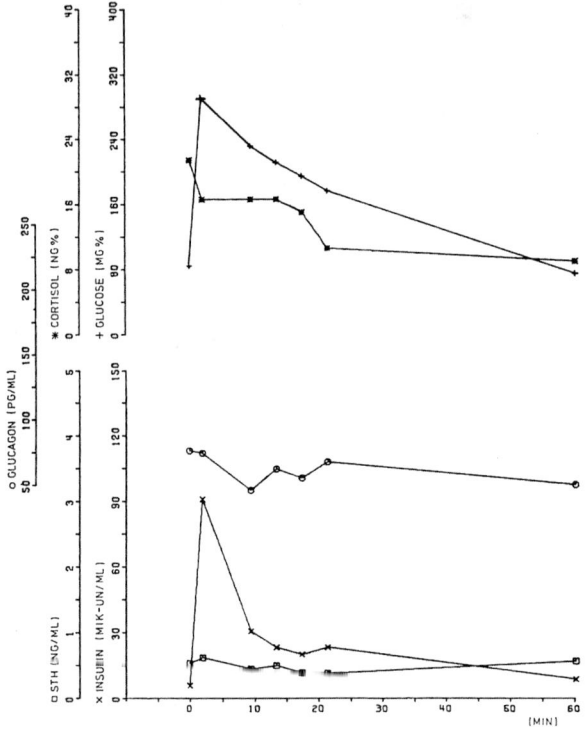

Fig. 26. Pattern of blood sugar, cortisol, insulin, HGH and glucagon in a healthy test subject of normal weight. Basal insulin level is below 10 μU/ml. First rise induced by glucose after two minutes up to 90 μU/ml, clearly marked second peak between 20 and 30 minutes, slightly raised cortisol sinks after glucose, basal HGH level unchanged, basal glucagon value 75 pg/ml, falling after glucose to 48 pg/ml

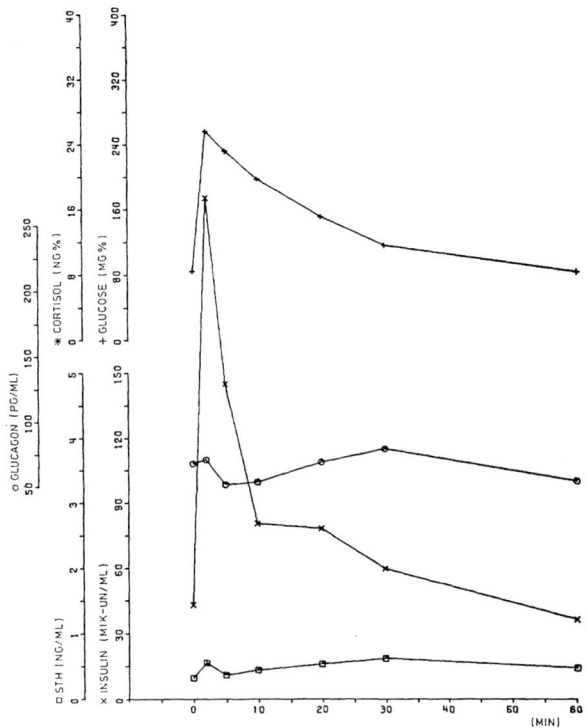

Fig. 27. Overweight normal subject; basal and glucose induced hyperinsulinaemia, basal glucagon 68 pg/ml, falling after i.v. glucose

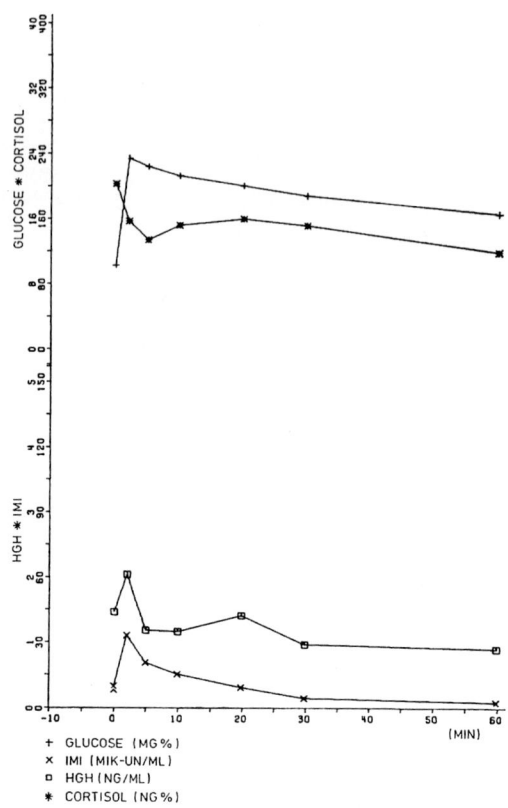

Fig. 28. Underweight fasting normal subject, basal insulin level very low, slight
rise induced by glucose, reactive rise of cortisol after 20 minutes

Whole Group

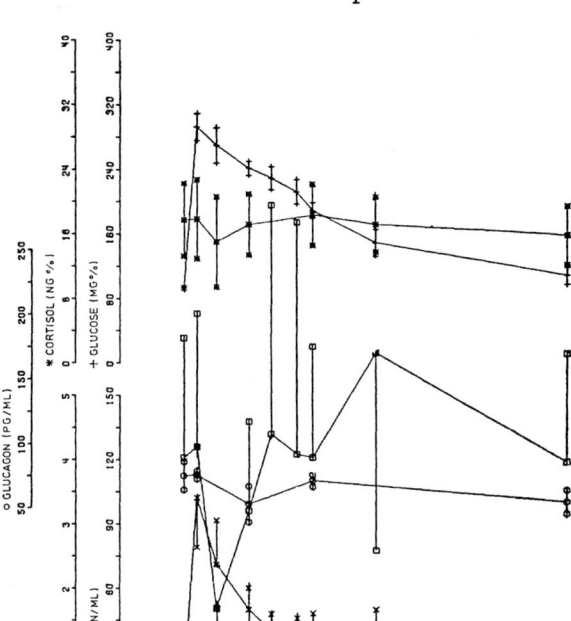

Fig. 29. Fasting blood sugar values 85 mg%, 60 minutes after the load has almost returned to the initial value. Average cortisol value 17 ng%, lowered by glucose after five to ten minutes. After 60 minutes it remains below the initial value. Average basal insulin concentration 14 µU/ml, two minutes after end of glucose injection, average values up to 95 µU/ml, well marked second peak after 20 minutes; after 60 minutes the initial concentration is almost reached. Average of HGH at 3.8 ng%, between the fifth and 18 minutes the initial value is reduced to one half by glucose, but is reached again after 60 minutes. Basal glucagon figures 61 pg/ml, dropping after i.v. glucose

Summary

Healthy subjects in relation to their body weight show striking fluctuations of basal and glucose-induced insulin levels which almost returned to the initial values 60 minutes after the glucose injection. HGH and cortisol fell with the glucose load but they reach the initial value after 60 minutes. Glucagon falls after glucose and still remains below the basal level, even after 60 minutes.

4.4.2. *Diabetics*

Individual Examples

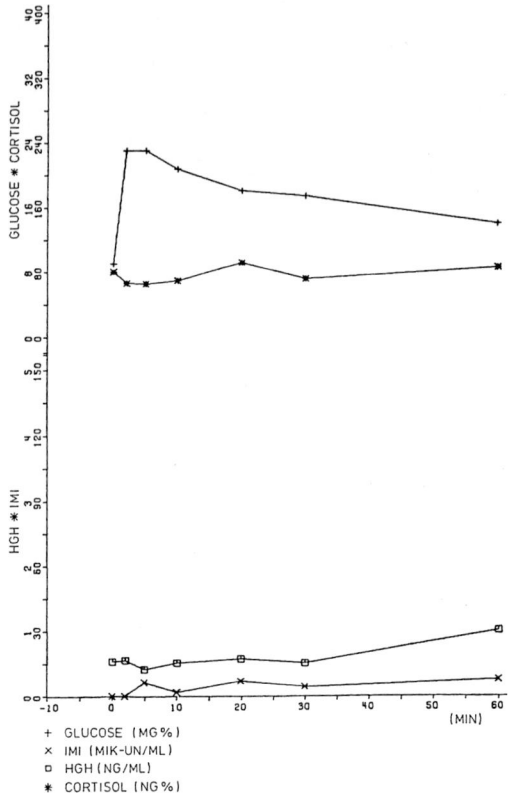

Fig. 30. Forty-year-old diabetic controlled by oral hypoglycaemic agents and diet; absent basal and very slight reactive insulin secretion, slight fall of cortisol, basal HGH secretion unchanged

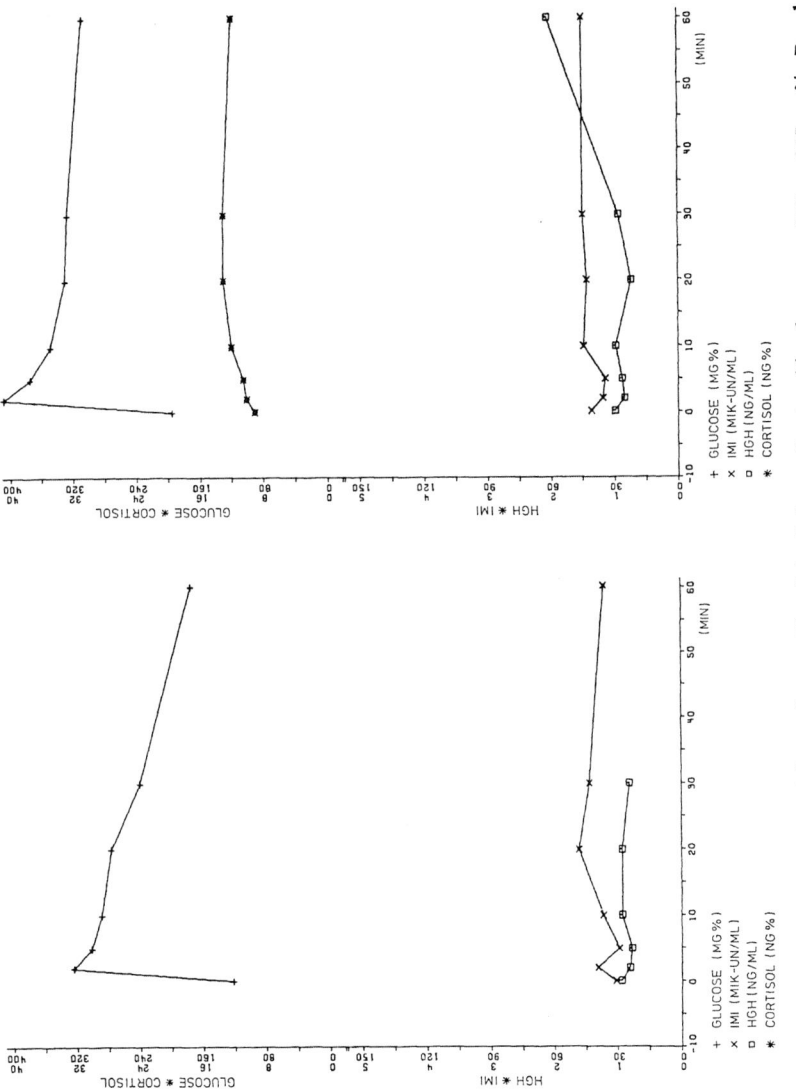

Figs. 31 and 32. Two overweight patients with adult diabetes. Fasting blood sugar at 120 to 195 mg%. Basal insulin raised but no additional output of insulin with glucose, paralysis of secretion, slight drop in HGH values

Whole Group

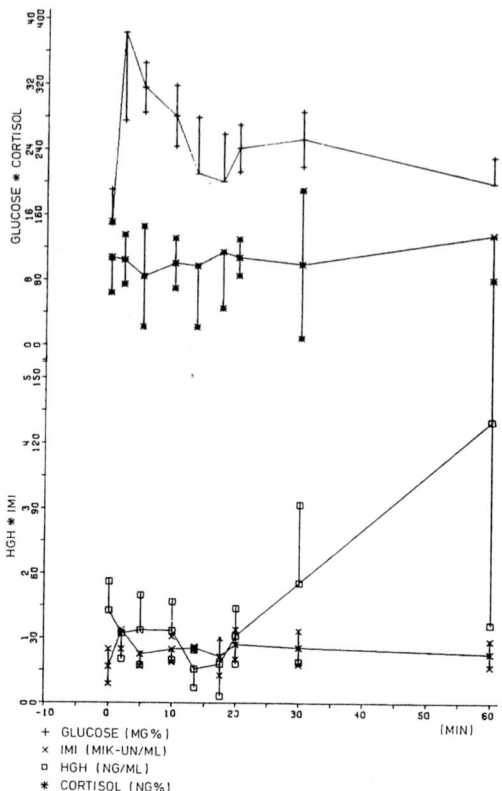

Fig. 33. Fasting blood sugar raised to an average of 145 mg%, one hour after glucose load the blood sugar reached 200 mg%. Cortisol at 10 ng% lower than in the healthy. The level is temporarily lowered by glucose. Basal HGH level at 1.4 ng/ml lower than in healthy (because of raised blood sugar), lowered to half the initial level by glucose. Insulin: only slight rise of basal levels of 15 µU/ml

Summary

Fasting blood sugar raised at 145 mg%, and still higher level after 60 minutes at 200 mg%. Cortisol at 10 ng% and HGH at 1.4 ng/ml definitely lower than in the healthy, lowered by i.v. glucose. Only a very slight rise of insulin induced by glucose.

4.4.3. All Intracranial Tumours

4.4.3 a. Pre-Operative

Individual Examples

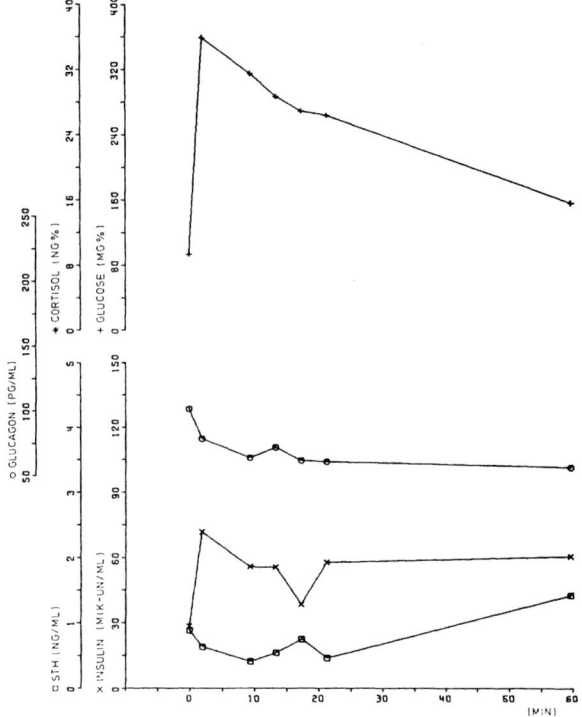

Fig. 34. Thirty-year-old patient with bifrontal cerebral tumour (butterfly glioma, astrocytoma Grade II). Normal blood sugar, slightly raised basal and normal glucose-induced secretion. HGH lowered by glucose. Fasting glucagon 102 pg/ml, definitely falling with i.v. glucose

Results

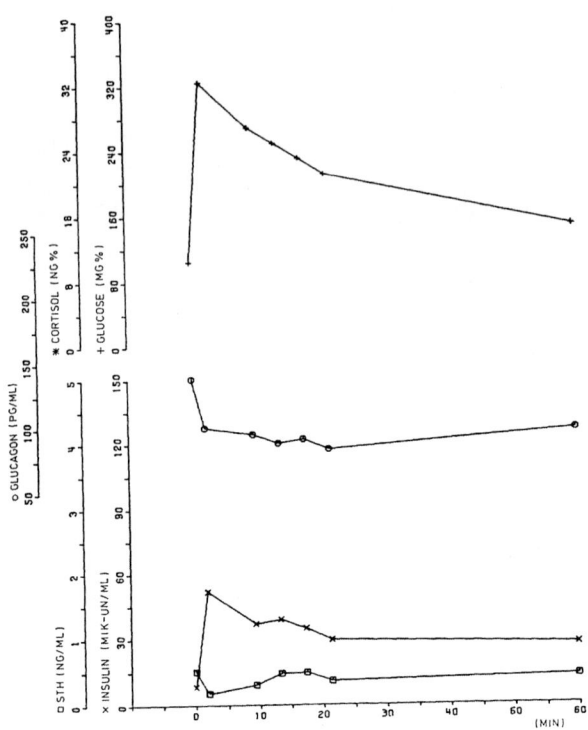

Fig. 35. Forty-five-year-old man with suprasellar chromophobe adenoma. Fasting glucose, basal and reactive insulin level normal. Basal HGH below 1 ng/ml, fasting glucagon 138 pg/ml but falling with i.v. glucose

Entire Group Pre-Operative

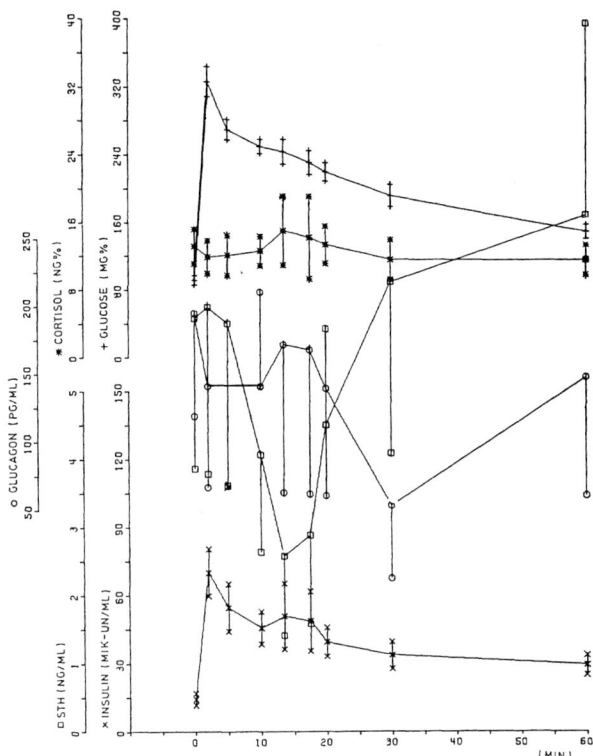

Fig. 36. Fasting blood sugar 85 mg%, as in the healthy subjects; after 60 minutes values still raised at 145 mg%. Cortisol with an average value of 13 ng%, is lower than in the healthy. Slight tendency to drop after glucose. Basal insulin level 15 μU/ml, mean value two minutes after end of injection 60 μU/ml, well marked second peak after 20 minutes. Mean HGH value at 5 ng/ml, level lowered by glucose. big fluctuations of the mean (acromegaly patients included in this group). Fasting glucagon level 194 pg/ml falling with intravenous glucose

Summary

Fasting blood sugar level as in the healthy, cortisol lower at 13 ng%, basal insulin as high as in the healthy. Glucose-induced rise definitely less than in the healthy. Glucagon slightly raised compared with the healthy, normal fall with intravenous glucose.

*4.4.3 b. First Post-Operative Day (Conscious Patients Free of
Complications)*

Individual Examples

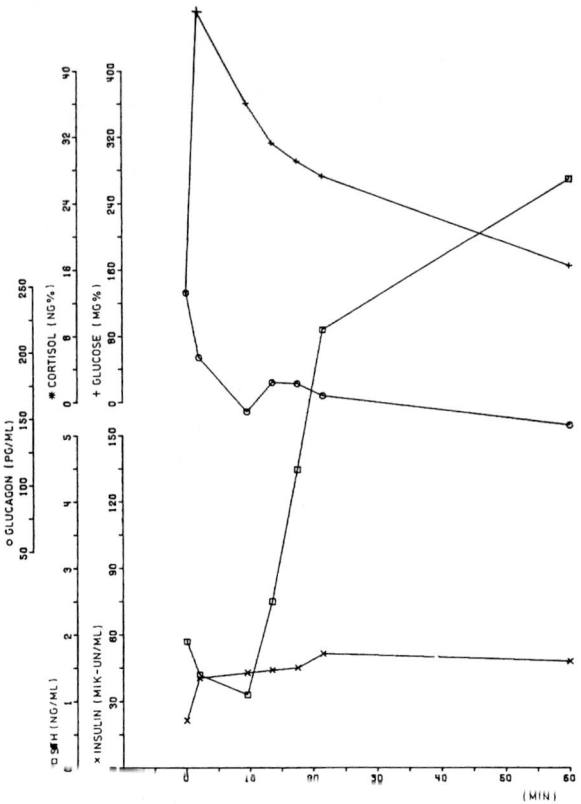

Fig. 37. Fasting blood sugar raised to 135 mg%, delayed rise of basal insulin with
intravenous glucose. Glucagon at 245 pg/ml definitely raised, but falling with
glucose

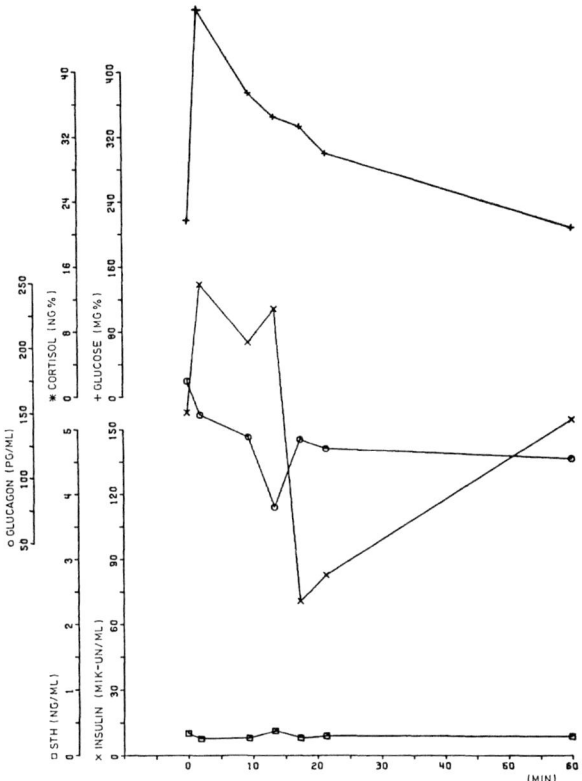

Fig. 38. Hyperglycaemia 210 mg⁰/o, marked basal hyperinsulinaemia, HGH shows basal values at 1 ng/ml, glucagon at 175 pg/ml definitely raised, showing physiological fall with i.v. glucose

Entire Group

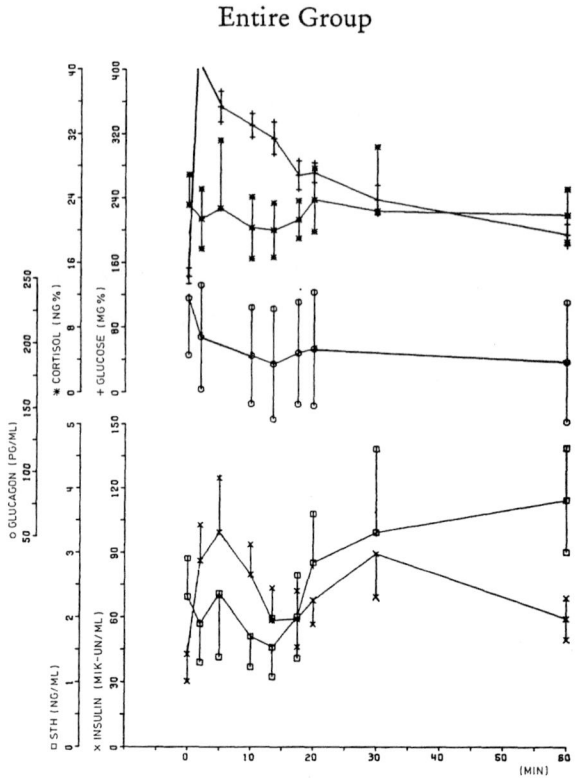

Fig. 39. Basal blood sugar level at 150 mg%, cortisol very definitely raised at 23 ng%, falling with glucose. Basal insulin raised at 45 µU/ml with a reactive rise after 5 minutes to 100 µU/ml. Second peak after 20 to 30 minutes (basal and glucose induced hyperinsulinaemia) HGH definitely lowered, compared with pre-operative, values further lowered by intravenous glucose. Basal glucagon definitely raised on the first post-operative day, falling with i.v. glucose

Summary

Hyperglycaemia at 150 mg%, cortisol raised at 23 ng%, HGH lowered, both falling with intravenous glucose. Marked basal and glucose-induced hyperinsulinaemia. Glucagon definitely raised, falling physiologically with i.v. glucose.

4.4.3 c. Seventh Post-Operative Day (Uncomplicated Pattern)

Individual Examples

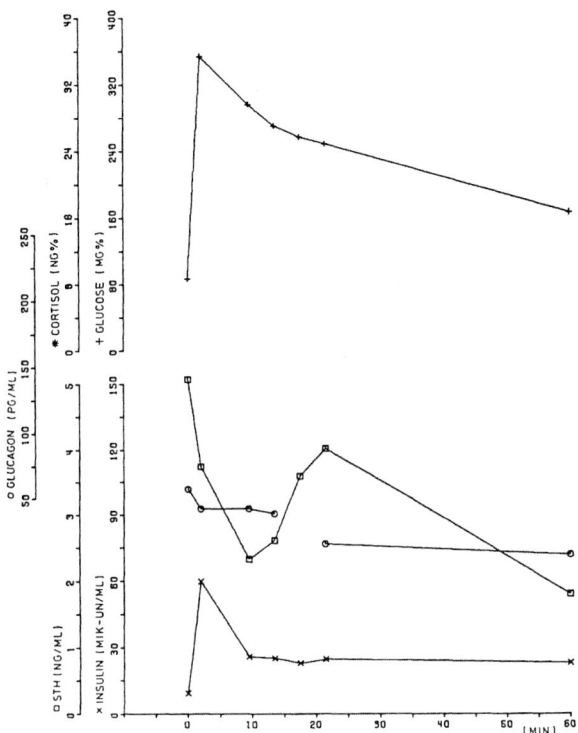

Fig. 40. Blood sugar at 95 mg⁰/o at upper limit of normal. Normal basal and glucose-induced insulin secretion. Glucagon at 57 pg/ml in lower normal range, falling with glucose

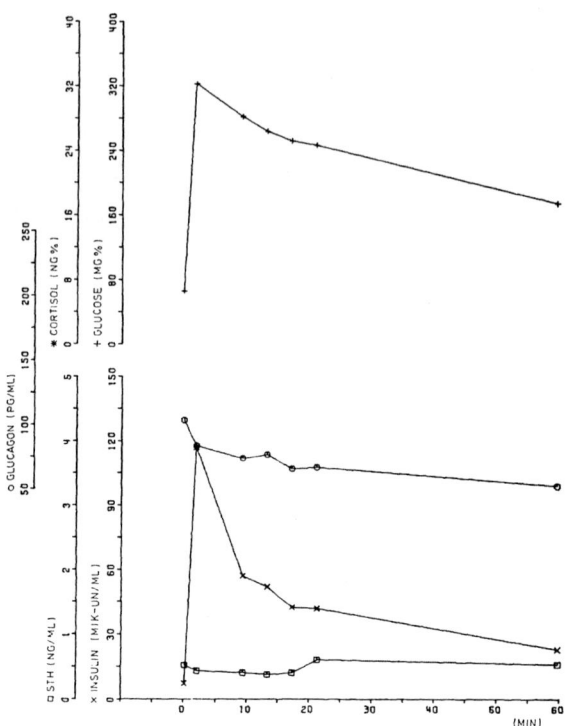

Fig. 41. Blood sugar within normal limits, normal basal and glucose-induced insulin secretion, HGH below 1 ng/ml. Basal glucagon within normal range at 103 pg/ml, falling further with glucose

Entire Group

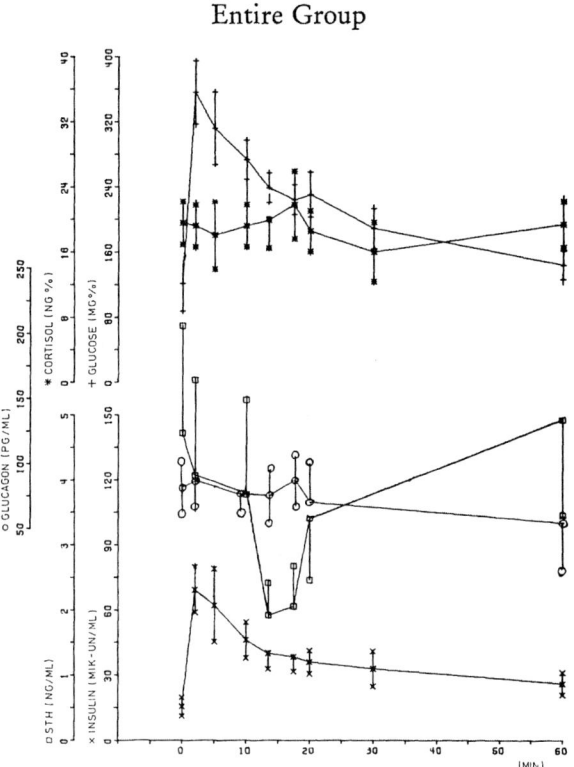

Fig. 42. Basal blood sugar raised at 130 mg%, cortisol raised at 19 ng%, but lower compared with first post-operative day. Insulin slightly raised with basal levels at 17 μU/ml, reactive level as pre-operatively at 65 μU/ml. HGH again raised and falling as pre-operatively. Glucagon falling with glucose as pre-operatively

Summary

Operation led to reversible disturbance of the metabolism of glucose and its hormones, regardless of the size, location and histology of the brain tumours. The fasting blood sugar rises from 85 mg% on the first post-operative day to 150 mg%, and even on the 7th day is still raised at 130 mg%. The pre-operative basal cortisol level, which is low compared with healthy subjects, climbs from 13 to 23 ng% and even on the 7th day it is still high at 19 ng%. The basal pre-operative insulin is normal, the glucose-induced insulin secretion slightly reduced in comparison with healthy subjects. On the first post-operative day a marked rise of the fasting level and the reactive values is observed (basal and reactive hyper-insulinaemia). On the 7th post-operative day the basal levels are only slightly raised and the glucose-induced insulinaemia corresponds to the pre-operative. On the first post-operative day, as might be expected, the HGH is low, as the acromegaly patients are included in this group of intracranial tumours. In comparison with the healthy, the basal glucagon is slightly raised pre-operatively. On the first post-operative day a marked rise of the secretion develops, which is still detectable on the 7th post-operative day.

The physiological drop with intravenous glucose is also apparent post-operatively.

The concentrations of all the substances enumerated (including HGH, see Group 4 and 8 without acromegaly) are raised on the first post-operative day and are falling by the 7th post-operative day towards the initial pre-operative value.

Post-operatively the physiological reaction to glucose persists at a raised level: a rise of insulin and drop in cortisol, HGH and glucagon.

4.4.4. Endocrine Inactive Intra- and Suprasellar Pituitary Tumours

4.4.4 a. Pre-Operative

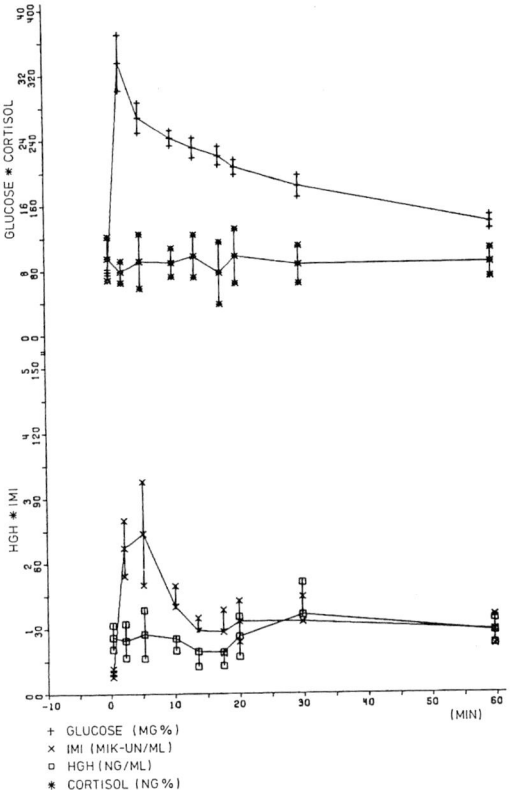

+ GLUCOSE (MG %)
× IMI (MIK-UN/ML)
□ HGH (NG/ML)
* CORTISOL (NG%)

Fig. 43. Low average blood sugar at 78 mg⁰/₀, low cortisol values without any change in response to glucose. Compared with the healthy and the total group of intracranial tumours the basal insulin is lower at 6–7 μU/ml; the first reactive insulin level up to 75 μU/ml, second peak by the 20th to 30th minute. Basal HGH values with little tendency to fall from the 10th to 20th minute

4.4.4 b. First Post-Operative Day

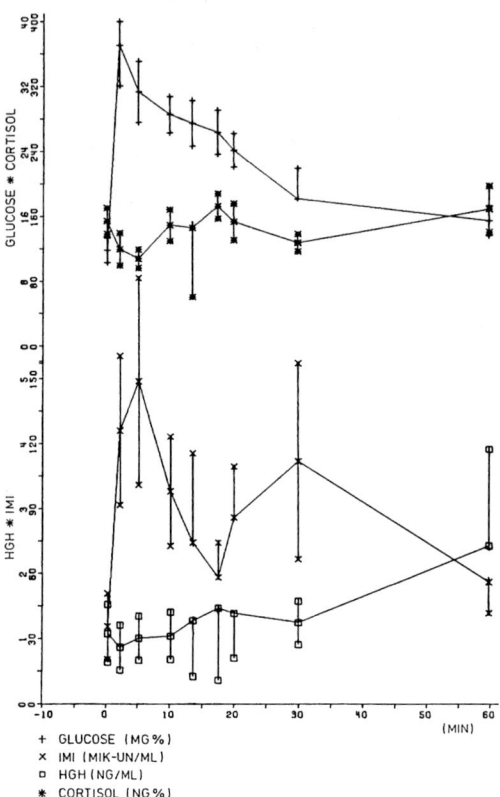

Fig. 44. Blood sugar at 130 mg⁰/o, cortisol raised at 15 ng⁰/o—this can be lowered by glucose. Basal hyperinsulinaemia at 40 μU/ml and marked reactive rise to 150 μU/ml. Second peak after 30 minutes, marked basal and glucose-induced hyper-insulinaemia. HGH basal values can be lowered only temporarily by glucose

4.4.4 c. Seventh Post-Operative Day

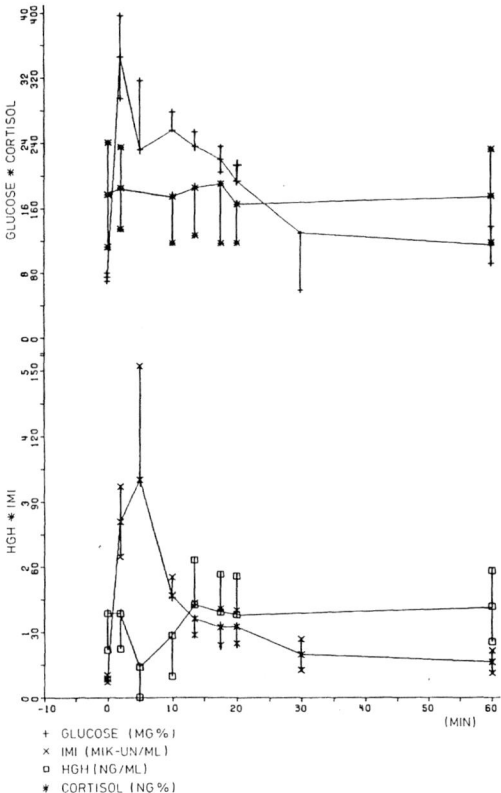

Fig. 45. Blood sugar at 76 mg%, as pre-operatively, basal insulin level low at 6 µU/ml, glucose-induced rise of insulin at 100 µU/ml still apparent after five minutes, raised compared with pre-operatively, but lower compared with values of the first post-operative day

Summary

The endocrinologically inactive pituitary tumours are distinguished from healthy subjects and the whole group of intracranial tumours by a lower fasting level for glucose and insulin and by a marked drop of HGH and cortisol, which show no clear cut reaction to intravenous glucose.

Post-operatively, on the first day there is, as in the whole group, a slightly less marked hyperglycaemia and a considerable basal and reactive hyperinsulinaemia, which is substantially greater than in the total group. The post-operative rise of cortisol and HGH is less marked or slight. On the seventh post-operative day the blood sugar and basal insulin are back to the pre-operative level, the glucose-induced insulin secretion has diminished, but the low pre-operative values have not yet been reached.

4.4.5. Endocrine Active Eosinophilic Adenomas with Pathological HGH Secretion

4.4.5 a. Pre-Operative

Individual Example

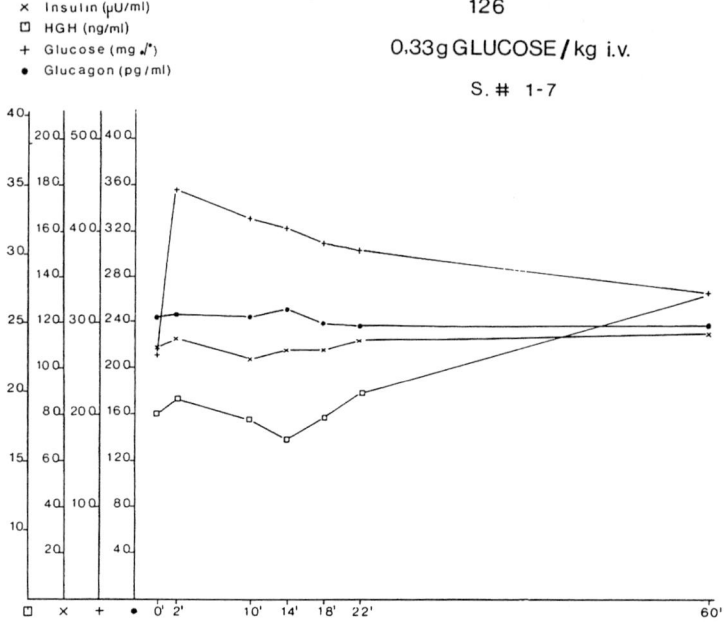

Fig. 46. 55-year-old woman, clinical signs of acromegaly for 20 years, diabetes mellitus requiring insulin for ten years (52 units depot insulin a.m. and 44 units depot insulin p.m.). Fasting blood sugar 210 mg%, basal insulin raised at 105 (!) μU/ml. No increase of secretion with glucose, but sustained secretion at this high level. HGH definitely raised at 18 ng/ml and no definite fall with glucose. Glucagon raised at 240 pg/ml, no drop with glucose

4.4.5 b. First Post-Operative Day (After Transnasal Trans-Sphenoidal Hypophysectomy)

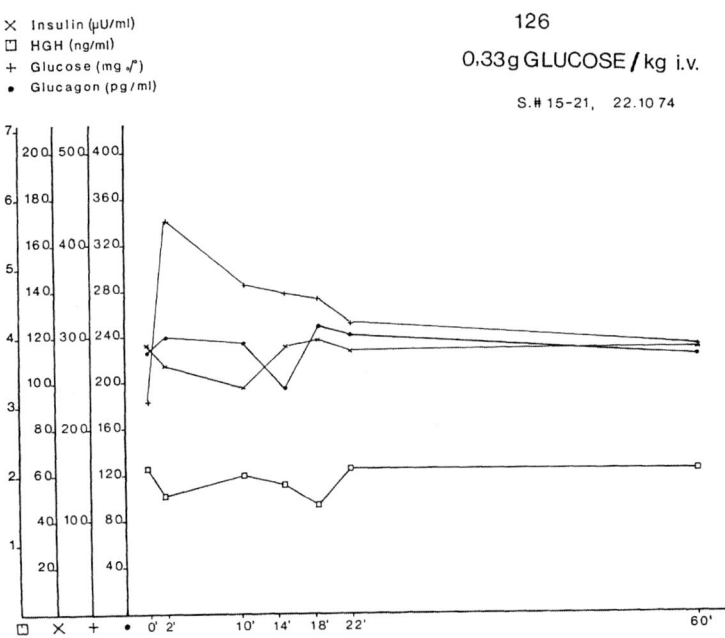

Fig. 47. Fasting blood sugar level 180 mg%, basal insulin secretion remaining high and showing no response to i.v. glucose. HGH in the normal range at 2 ng/ml, possibly a hint of a drop with glucose. Persistent high glucagon secretion and no fall with glucose

4.4.5 c. Seventh Post-Operative Day

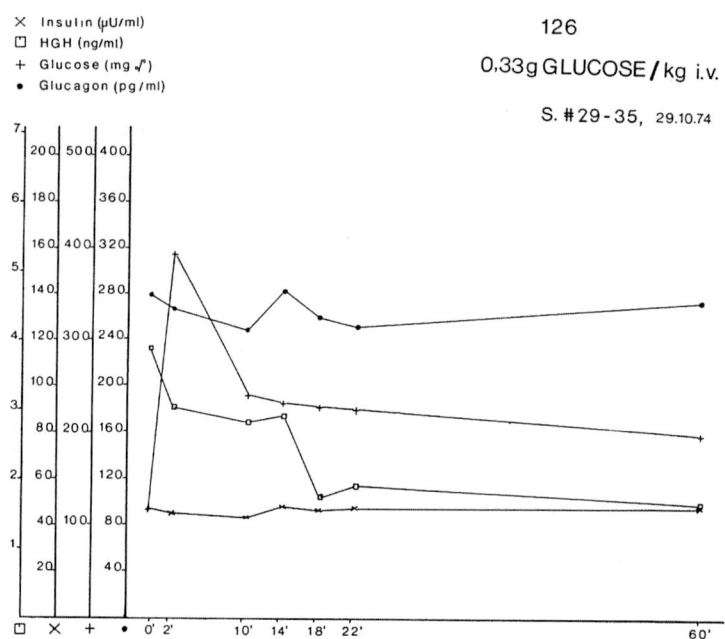

× Insulin (µU/ml)
☐ HGH (ng/ml)
+ Glucose (mg ‰)
• Glucagon (pg/ml)

126

0,33g GLUCOSE / kg i.v.

S. # 29 - 35, 29.10.74

Fig. 48. Fasting blood sugar at 120 mg⁰/₀. Basal insulin secretion at 45 µU/ml, very definitely lower. Also no glucose-induced rise. HGH at 3.8 ng/ml fell to under 2 ng/ml with intravenous glucose. The secretion of glucagon remained high and was not lowered by glucose. Dramatic drop in the insulin requirement. With a single dose of 16 units of depot insulin the daily profile of blood sugar values was 119, 225, and 135 mg⁰/₀. Mean concentration of blood sugar, HGH, cortisol and insulin in the whole group of acromegalics are shown in Figs. 83, 84, 85, and 86

4.4.6. Patients with Complete Anterior Pituitary Failure

Individual Examples

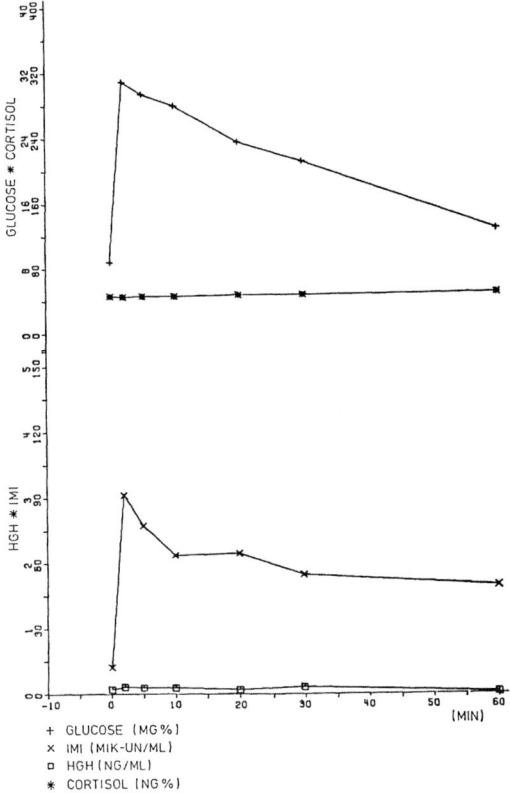

Fig. 49. 48-year-old patient with chromophobe adenoma, clinical and endocrinological evidence of complete anterior pituitary failure. Normal behaviour of blood sugar and insulin secretion, no reaction to glucose at low basal cortisol levels and no HGH

Whole Group

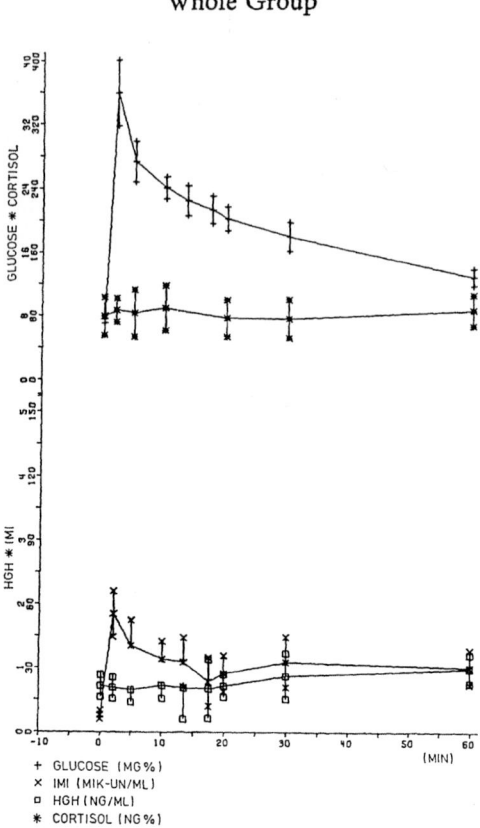

Fig. 50. Fasting blood sugar level at 76 mg⁰/o. Cortisol level low at 8 ng⁰/o, and no reaction to glucose. Basal insulin level at 6 μU/ml, glucose-induced secretion at 50 μU/ml, with a hint of a peak from the 20th to the 30th minute, very low HGH level at 0.7 ng⁰/o

Summary

In patients with complete anterior pituitary failure the fasting blood sugar and basal insulin concentrations are as low as in the inactive pituitary tumours, in comparison with this group, glucose-induced insulin secretion is still less. Cortisol and HGH show basal levels without any response to glucose.

4.4.7. Para-Hypothalamic Tumours with Mechanical Changes, Displacement and Chronic Damage

4.4.7 a. Pre-Operative

Individual Examples

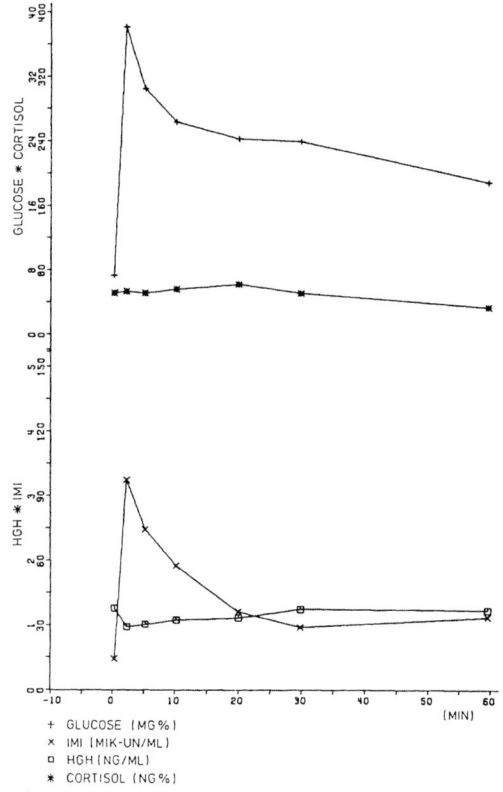

Fig. 51. Bilateral olfactory groove meningioma, in a 50-year-old man, which had led to marked dorsal displacement of the third ventricle and the hypothalamus. Normal fasting blood sugar, normal basal and reactive insulin secretion, basal cortisol level, normal HGH with slight inhibition of secretion by glucose

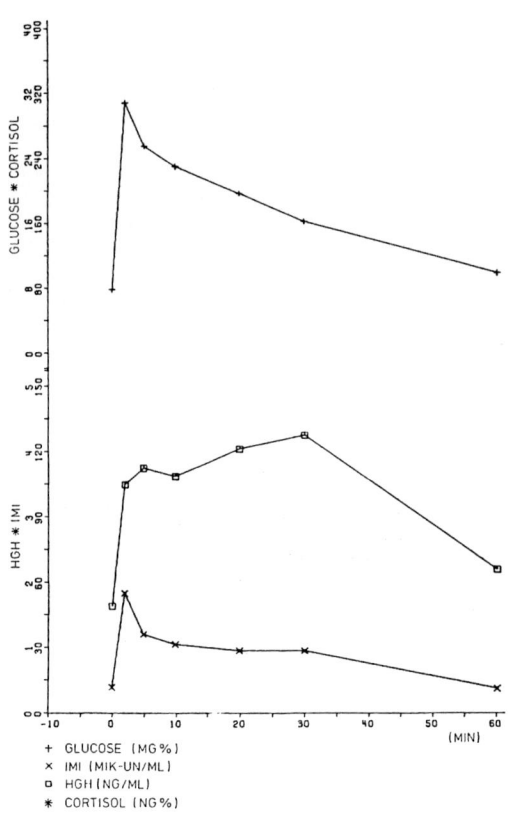

Fig. 52. Seven-year-old girl with optic nerve glioma (histology spongioblastoma Grade II) which had led to displacement of the pituitary stalk and the tuber cinereum. Nothing of note endocrinologically, normal insulin secretion, paradoxical rise of HGH with glucose, fasting blood sugar normal

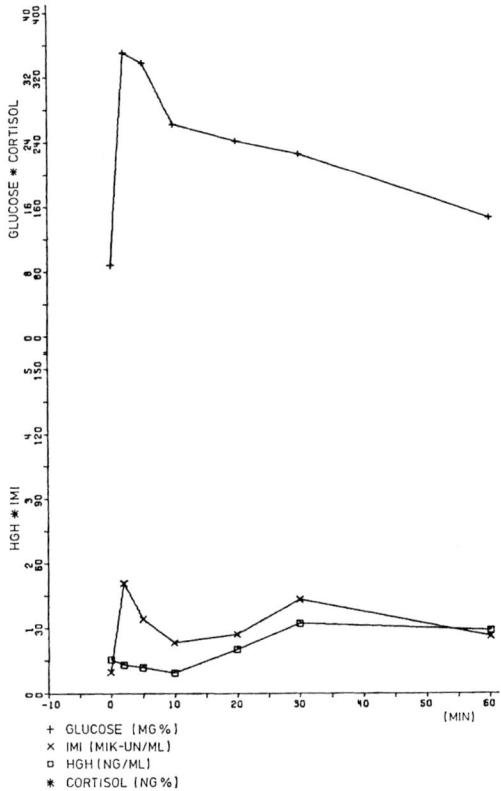

+ GLUCOSE (MG%)
× IMI (MIK-UN/ML)
□ HGH (NG/ML)
* CORTISOL (NG%)

Fig. 53. Seventeen-year-old patient with clinical and endocrinologically confirmed Frölich's syndrome (four year history, loss of vision, slight diabetes insipidus; histologically an astrocytoma of the diencephalon-stereotactic operation): normal basal and glucose-induced secretion, second peak at about the thirtieth minute, fasting blood sugar normal. HGH basal with values still falling slightly with glucose

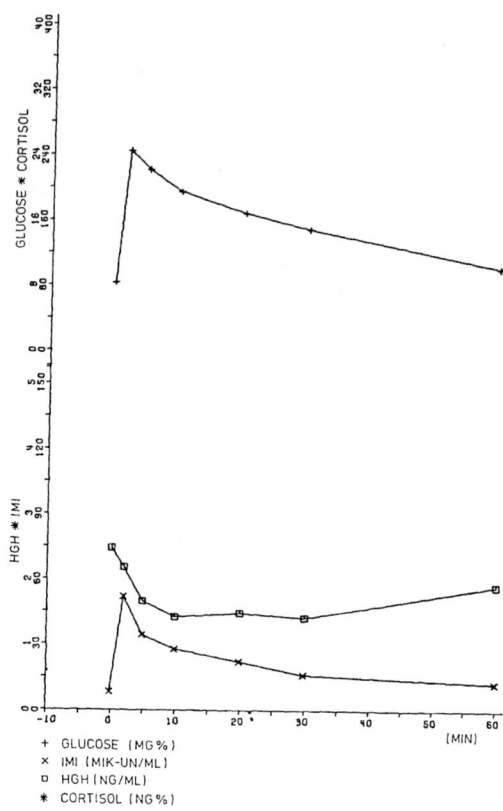

Fig. 54. Nine-year-old girl with clinical pubertas praecox associated with infantile obstructive hydrocephalus, the result of an aqueduct stenosis. Otherwise normal endocrine findings, normal HGH and cortisol response to insulin hypoglycaemia and arginine stress. Normal insulin secretion and prompt fall of HGH with glucose

Whole Group

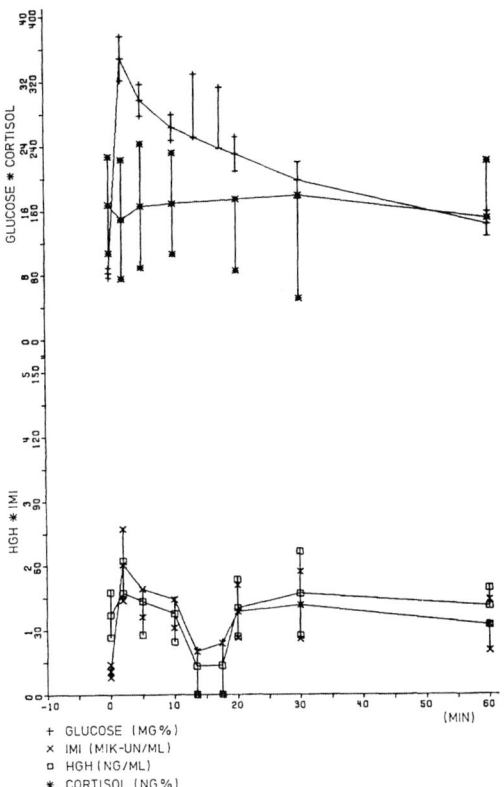

+ GLUCOSE (MG%)
× IMI (MIK-UN/ML)
□ HGH (NG/ML)
* CORTISOL (NG%)

Fig. 55. Basal blood sugar 80 mg⁰/₀, cortisol 16 to 17 ng⁰/₀, not lowered by glucose. Basal insulin level at 10 µU/ml lower than in the healthy. Glucose induced rise to 60 µU/ml, second peak in 20 to 30 minutes, HGH values low, and lowered to half the initial value by glucose, from the 10th to 20th minute

Summary

Even very extensive, chronically progressive tumours in the region of the hypothalamus do not lead to a disturbance of glucose metabolism in the direction of a hyperglycaemia. On the contrary the basal blood sugar and insulin level are low. There are not usually any hormone deficiencies and regulation is frequently intact (drop in HGH and cortisol with glucose, rise with arginine and insulin hypoglycaemia). The control mechanism for particular functions can be deranged without other endocrine abnormalities being apparent (pubertas praecox, paradoxical HGH rise with glucose).

4.4.7 b. First Post-Operative Day

Individual Examples

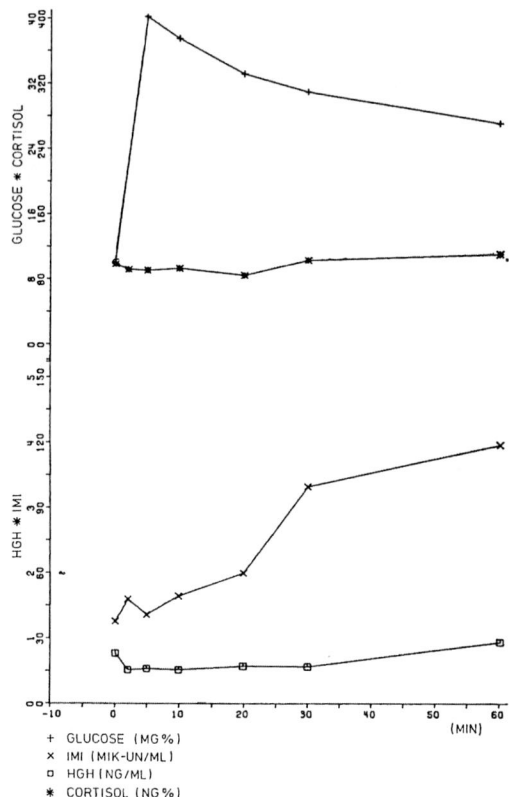

Fig. 56. In spite of a normal blood sugar, marked increase in basal insulin one day after operation on a craniopharyngioma in a 30-year-old patient. Delayed, then sustained glucose-induced rise of insulin. Cortisol and HGH at a low level showing a tendency to fall with glucose

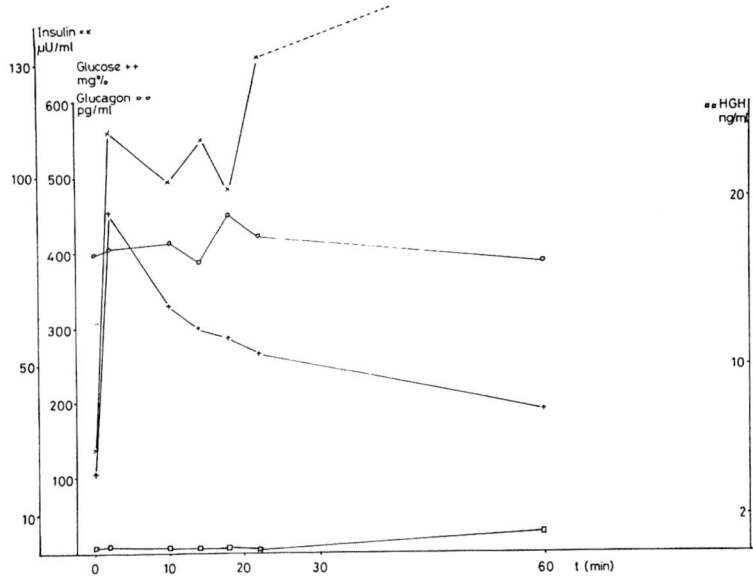

Fig. 57. Fifty-four-year-old patient with bilateral olfactory groove meningioma, uneventful progress, fully conscious. Raised basal insulin level with normal blood sugar and striking, sustained rise of insulin (hyperinsulinaemia) induced by glucose. Marked rise of basal glucagon at 397 pg/ml and no fall with glucose

Whole Group

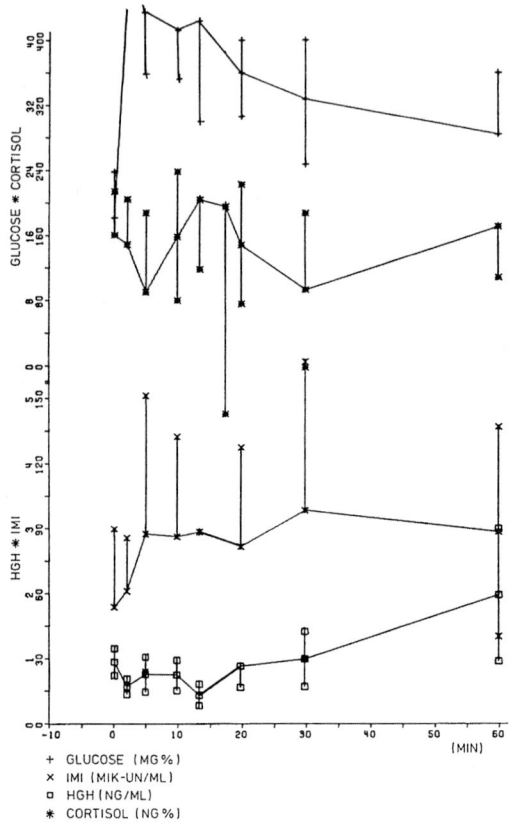

Fig. 58. Rise of fasting blood sugar level to 180 mg%, marked hyperglycaemia after intravenous glucose load. Cortisol values at 16 ng%, transitorily lowered with glucose. Striking basal hyperinsulinaemia at 52 µU/ml reactive rise with glucose to 90 µU/ml and this concentration had not even dropped again in 60 minutes. HGH levels—basal

It was not possible to establish a group of patients on the seventh post-operative day with tumours in the vicinity of the hypothalamus. On the one hand there is a higher mortality after operations on such tumours, and on the other there are prominent peripheral problems with the survivors such as respiratory, circulatory and renal failure, which interfere with a purposeful investigation of glucose metabolism. Individual examples can be seen in the account of the mean concentrations.

Summary

Brain tumours with mechanical changes, displacement and chronic damage of the hypothalamus show the following special features on the first post-operative day compared with the other post-operative groups: The fasting blood sugar is distinctly raised at 180 mg% and the fall in level after i.v. stress takes place more slowly (see also under Pharmacokinetics). The basal insulin concentration is raised and the secretion induced by glucose shows a change in pattern; the rise is delayed, climbing less obviously over the raised basal level, however the insulin secretion then persists at a high level and even after 60 minutes does not fall. The basal glucagon concentrations (individual cases) are raised compared with the total group of intracranial tumours. HGH and cortisol are reduced as compared with the total group and with the patients with cerebral hemisphere tumours.

4.4.8. Patients with Hemisphere Tumours Close to the Cortex

4.4.8 a. Pre-Operative

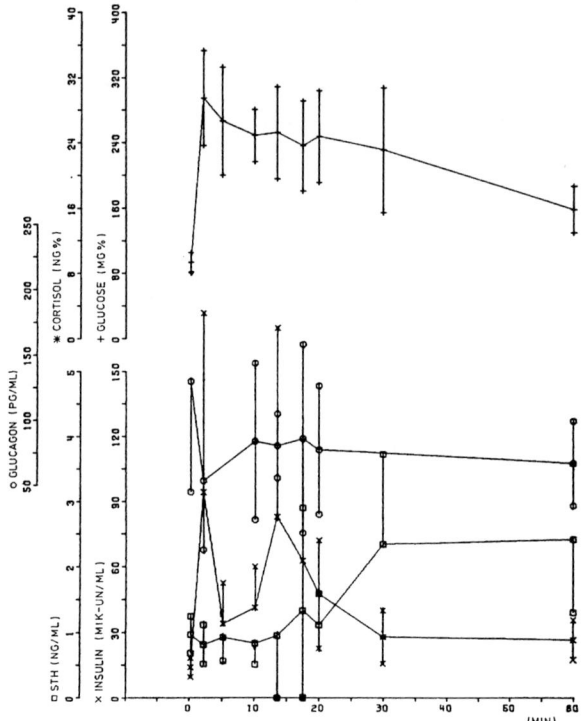

Fig. 59. Fasting values for blood sugar and insulin are normal at 90 mg% and 13 µU/ml respectively. After 60 minutes blood sugar still remains at 160 mg%. Glucose-induced rise of insulin shows two peaks with quite a marked scatter. After 60 minutes, the fasting level is almost attained. HGH less than 1 ng/ml— tendency to drop with glucose. A slight rise commences at the 18th minute up to 2.3 ng/ml in the 60th minute. Glucagon at 130 pg/ml is definitely raised compared with the healthy and falls with intravenous glucose

4.4.8 b. First Post-Operative Day

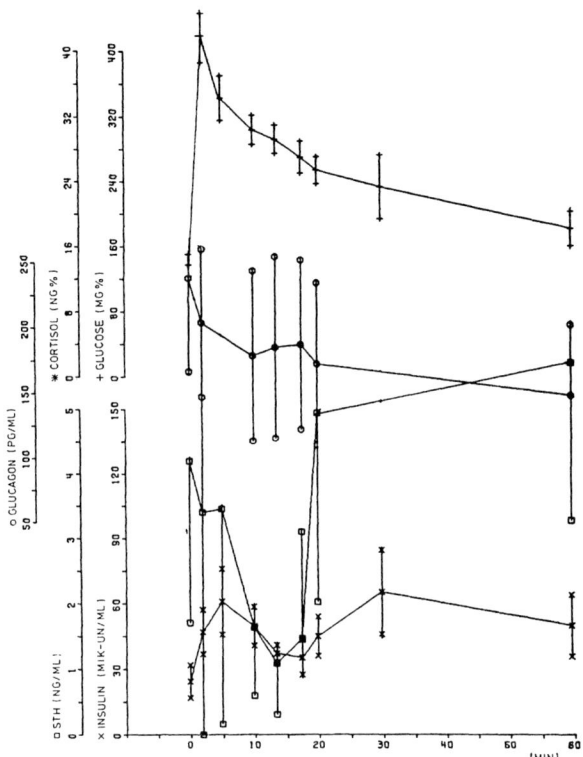

Fig. 60. Fasting concentrations raised at 140 mg⁰/o and after 60 minutes still high values of 180 mg⁰/o. Fasting insulin level raised at 25 µU/ml, delayed biphasic rise with glucose up to 60 µU/ml, HGH raised to 4.2 ng/ml, steep fall with glucose up to the 14th minute, then a quicker rise to just over the initial value. Glucagon at 237 pg/ml markedly raised compared with pre-operatively, and a physiological fall with glucose

4.4.8 c. Seventh Post-Operative Day

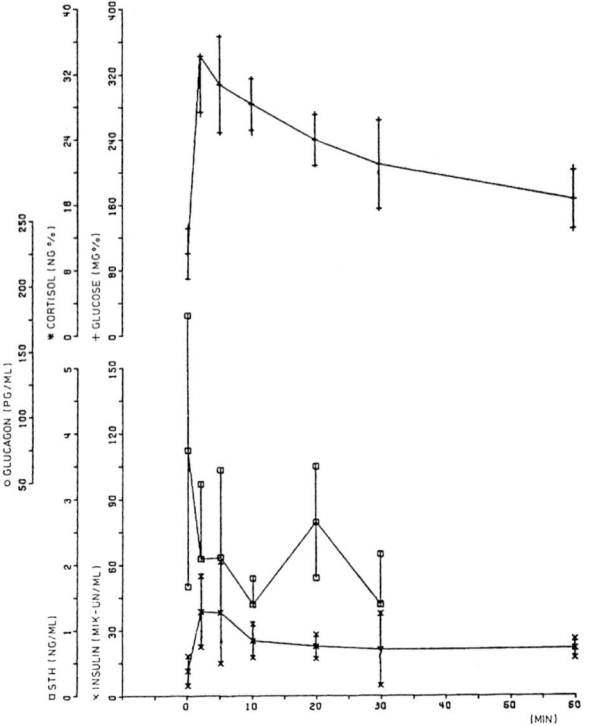

Fig. 61. Fasting blood sugar slightly raised at 103 mg/ml, after 60 minutes there is a level of 160 mg%. Basal insulin in the normal range with moderate rise induced by glucose. HGH at 3.7 ng/ml still raised, quicker fall with glucose

Summary

Compared with healthy subjects superficial cortical hemisphere tumours show normal fasting values for blood sugar and pre-operative insulin. HGH is significantly lower. Glucagon is definitely raised. The operation leads on the first day to a rise of all values with preservation of the physiological reaction to glucose (rise of insulin, fall of the raised level of HGH and glucagon). On the seventh day the blood sugar and HGH show a downward tendency but have still not reached the pre-operative values. Basal and reactive insulin levels are low normal.

4.4.9. Unconscious Patients with Acute "Midbrain Syndrome"

Individual Examples

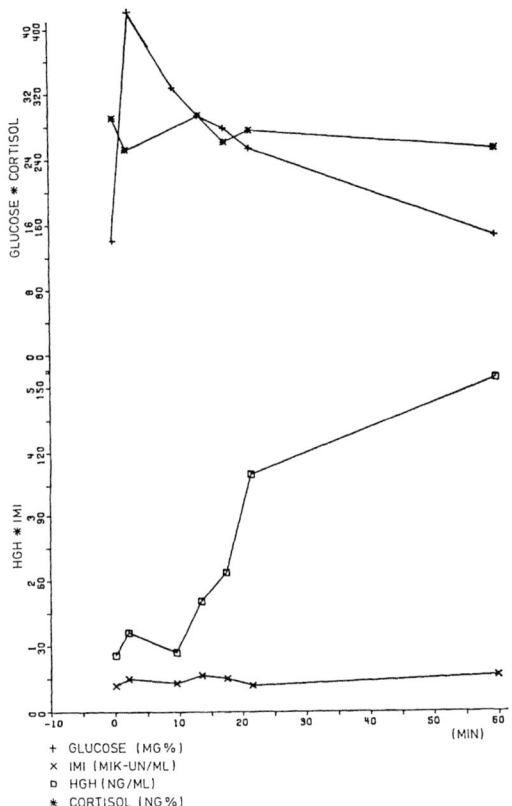

+ GLUCOSE (MG%)
× IMI (MIK-UN/ML)
□ HGH (NG/ML)
∗ CORTISOL (NG%)

Fig. 62. Thirty-year-old man, with fully developed picture of primary midbrain decerebration, after a severe closed craniocerebral injury. Investigations a few hours after the injury. Blood sugar 140 mg%, high cortisol secretion, basal insulin secretion normal, but none induced by glucose. Steeper rise of HGH with the commencing fall in blood sugar after i.v. bolus although the blood sugar was still between 200 and 300 mg%

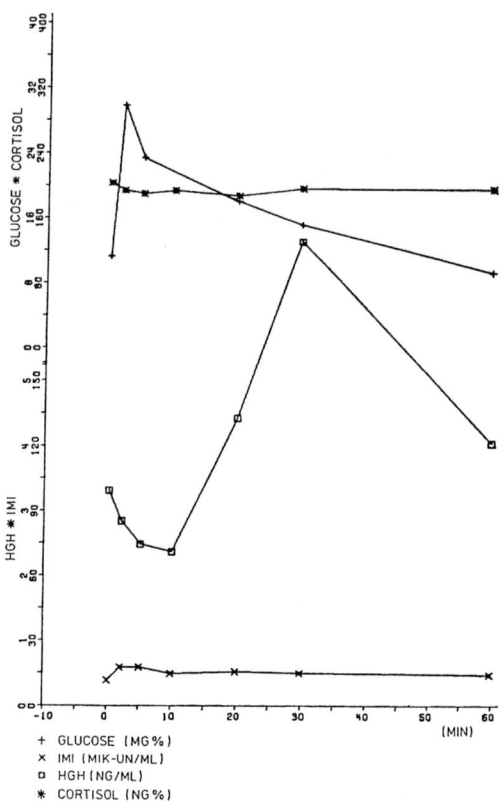

Fig. 63. Sixty-two-year old patient after a head injury without primary brain damage, acute subdural haematoma. Pre-operative mid-brain decerebration in transitional stage to bulbar damage. Post-operatively full picture of midbrain decerebration. Investigation hours after the operation Cortisol distinctly raised, normal basal insulin secretion but very little induced by glucose. Steep rise of HGH with high glucose levels after i.v. loading

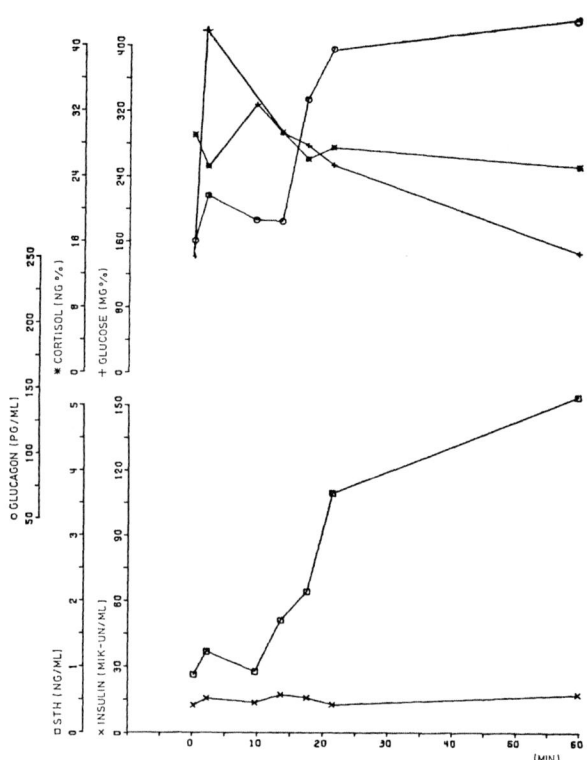

Fig. 64. Thirty-one-year old man, investigated a few hours after a severe cranio-cerebral injury. Clinically the full picture of a primary midbrain decerebration; moderate hyperglycaemia, high cortisol level, normal basal insulin secretion, but none induced by glucose. Paradoxical rise of HGH during fall of blood sugar within the hyperglycaemic range. Glucagon values raised at 260 pg% before the stress and pathological rise of concentration with glucose load

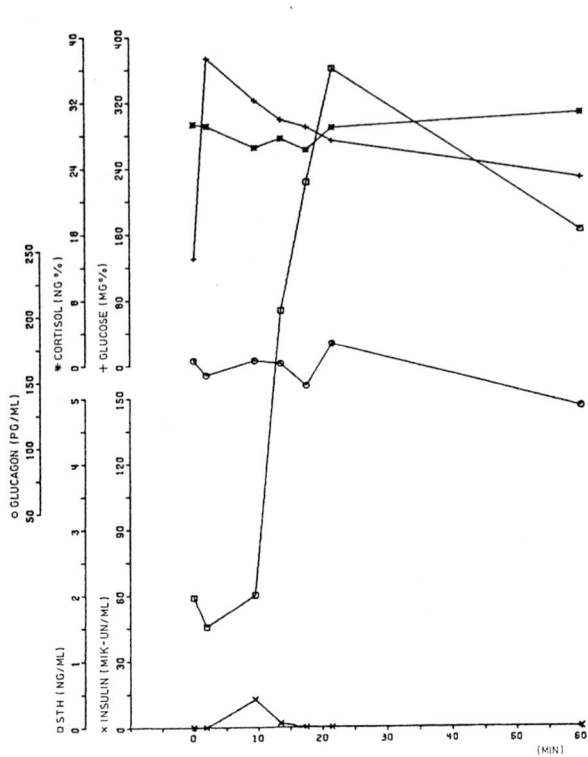

Fig. 65. Six hours after a severe craniocerebral injury moderate hyperglycaemia
of 130 mg⁰/o, very definitely raised cortisol secretion, absent basal insulin secretion
and only very slight secretion induced by glucose. Markedly steep rise in HGH
with a fall in blood sugar in the hyperglycaemic range, after intravenous stress.
Basal glucagon at 166 pg/ml definitely raised. Only slight fall with intravenous
glucose

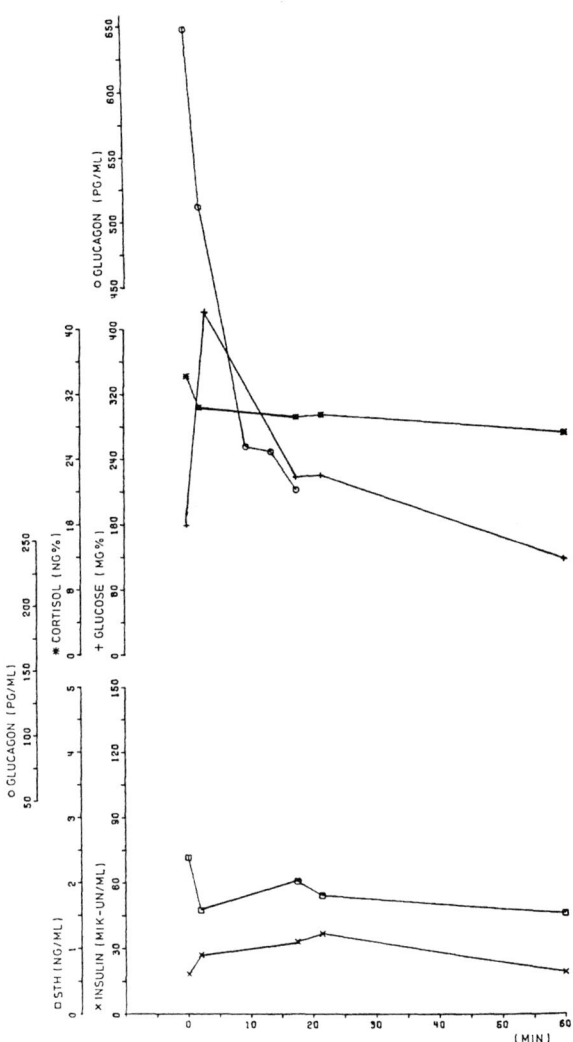

Fig. 66. Control investigations of this patient 24 hours later. Neurological findings unchanged: furthermore a high cortisol level and slight fall with glucose, moderate basal hyperglycaemia, basal insulin level slightly raised, smaller rise with glucose. HGH in the normal range. Basal glucagon levels markedly raised at 647 pg/ml, falling promptly with i.v. glucose

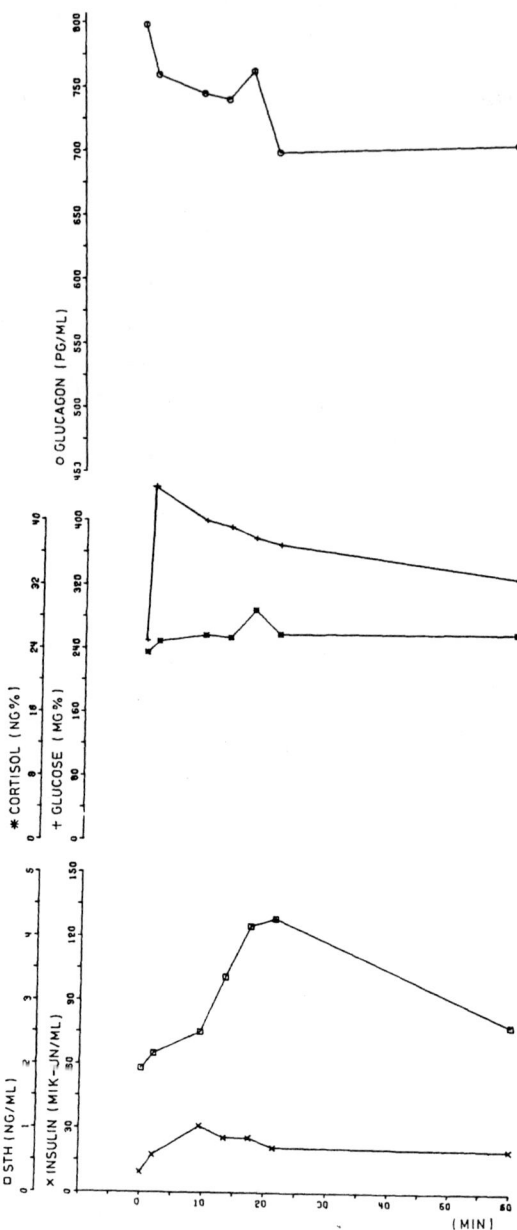

Fig. 67. Control investigations seven days after the injury. At the time of the transition of the clinical picture into a pontobulbar lesion: definite hyperglycaemia of 240 mg⁰/o, cortisol level still markedly raised, basal and glucose-induced insulin secretion unchanged. Paradoxical rise in HGH similar to the behaviour hours after the injury. Basal glucagon level excessively raised at 797 pg/ml and only a slight fall with i.v. glucose

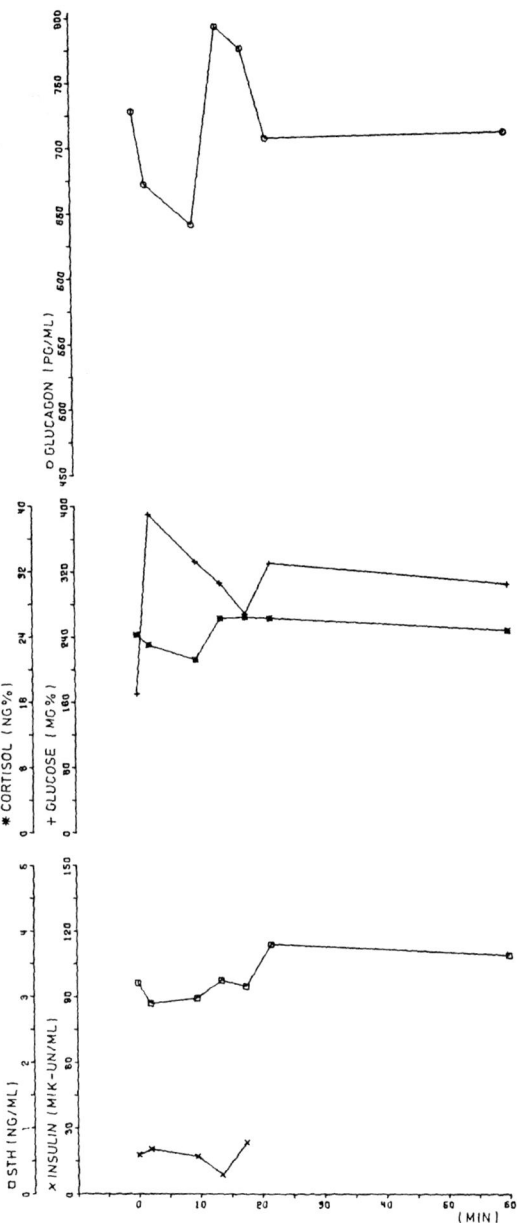

Fig. 68. Further examination three days later with clinical findings unchanged: Slightly raised basal, but absent glucose-induced insulin secretion. Normal HGH and raised cortisol level with a tendency to fall with flucose. Furthermore glucagon secretion maximally raised with basal level at 728 pg/ml but no sustained fall with i.v. glucose

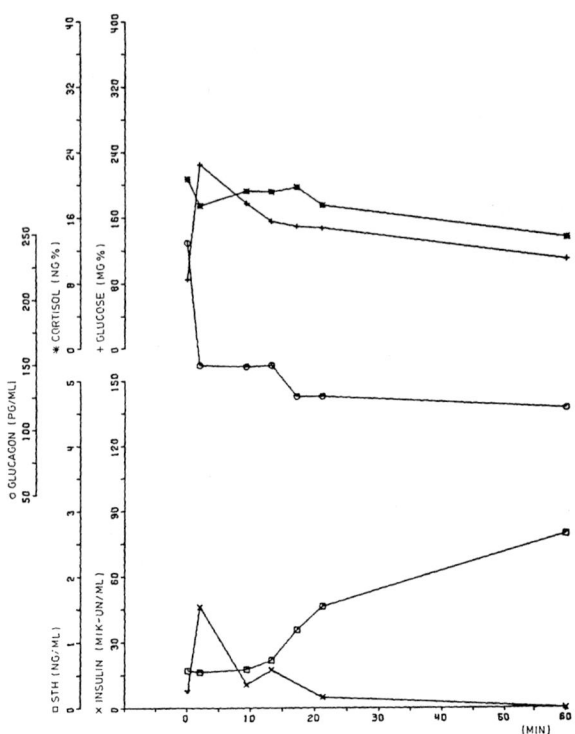

Fig. 69. Investigation 16 days later. Patient showed signs of the apallic state. Blood sugar normal, cortisol at 21 ng% still high, but now lower compared with the earlier investigations. Normal basal insulin secretion and almost normal glucose-induced secretion, sligher paradoxical rise of HGH with glucose. Basal glucagon still clearly raised and prompter fall with intravenous glucose into the upper range of normal

Total Group

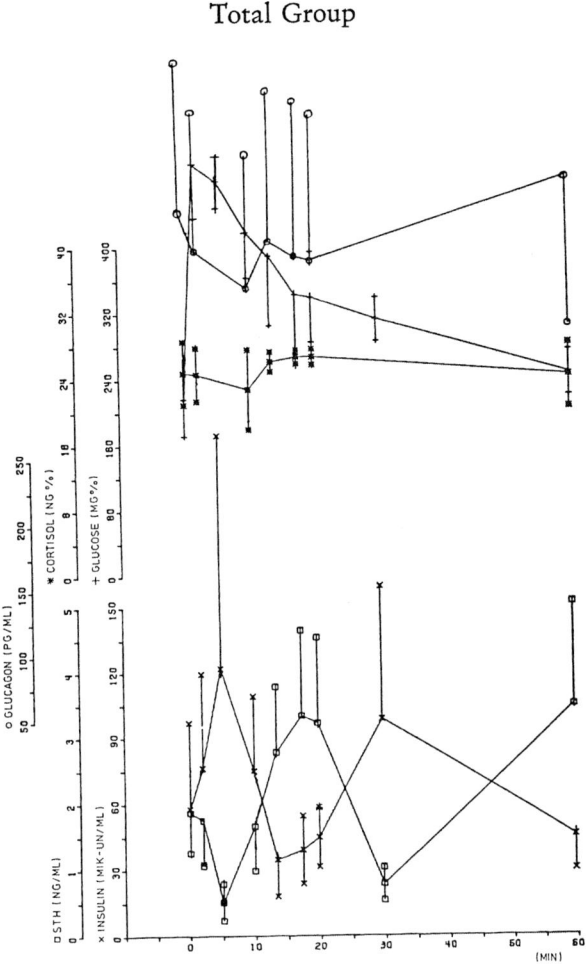

Fig. 70. Fasting hyperglycaemia at 210 mg%, increased assimilation of glucose after intravenous load (see also: Pharmacokinetics). Initial blood sugar values almost reached after 60 minutes. Cortisol raised to 26 ng%, only transitorily falling with glucose. Considerably raised basal insulin level at 75 µU/ml, with glucose a further rise of insulin concentration after five minutes to 120 µU/ml, then a steep fall and second peak near the 30th minute. After 60 minutes the basal values are still not attained. HGH in the normal range but with i.v. glucose, a paradoxical rise with the incipient fall of the glucose level in the hyperglycaemic range. Basal glucagon level excessively raised, only minimal fall with i.v. glucose

Summary

In comparison with the post-operative groups the fasting blood sugar, cortisol, basal insulin and glucagon are stimulated the greatest or maximum in those patients with an acute midbrain syndrome. In addition, the kinetics of the patterns of concentration are changed.

HGH shows a paradoxical steep rise five to ten minutes after intravenous glucose, while the blood sugar, which is still in the hyperglycaemic range, falls. This fall, *i.e.* the assimilation, is greatest in this group (see also Pharmacokinetics). The excessively raised glucagon does not definitely and/or permanently drop with i.v. glucose. The extremely high basal values of insulin secretion show only negligible further stimulation by intravenous glucose. The concentration falls in the 14th to the 22nd minute and after sixty minutes is below the basal value.

4.4.10. Unconscious Patients with Acute Mesencephalo-Ponto-Bulbar Lesions

Individual Example

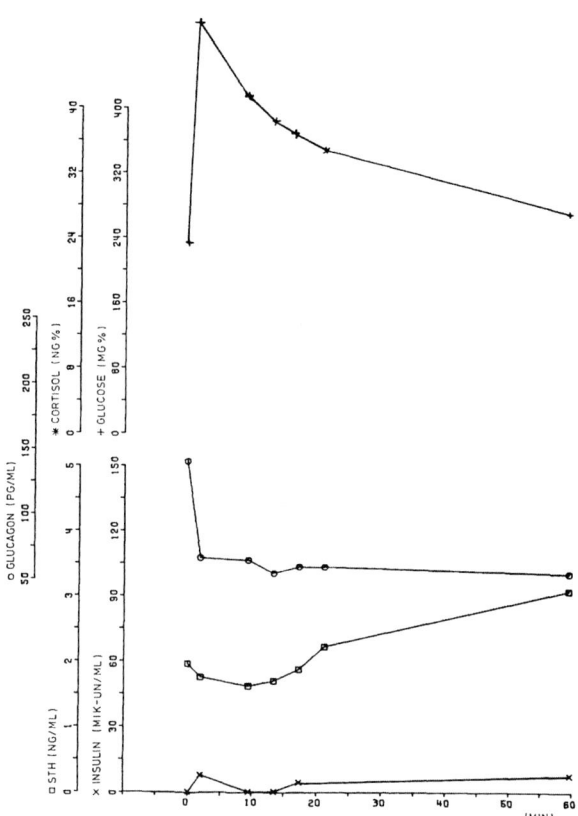

Fig. 71. A fourteen-year-old youth, mass bleeding in a recurrence of a cerebellar astrocytoma. Acute mesencephalo-ponto-bulbar syndrome. Raised blood sugar of 235 mg%. Basal insulin absent and only very minimal reactive secretion. HGH slight tendency to fall with glucose. Basal glucagon high normal, coming down into the normal range with intravenous glucose

Whole Group

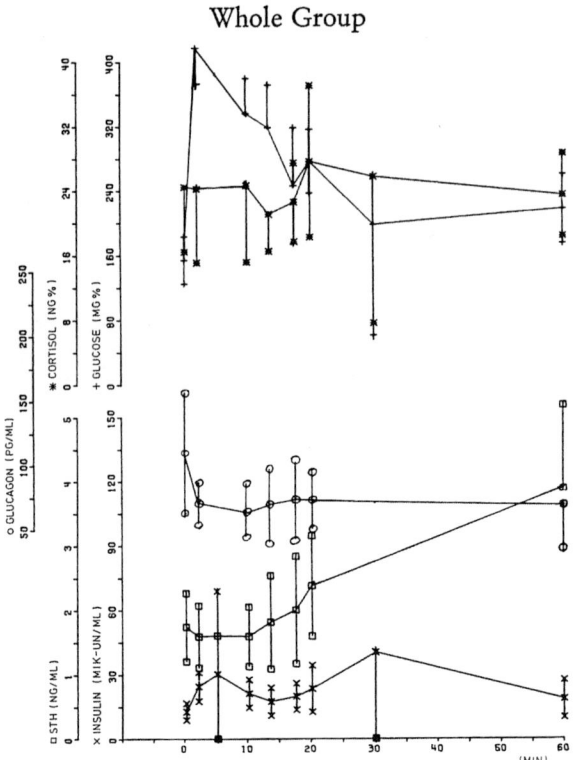

Fig. 72. Rise of blood sugar to 156 mg%. High cortisol levels at 25 ng%. Basal insulin level normal at 12 μU/ml. Only very slight biphasic rise with intravenous glucose after five and thirty minutes. HGH in normal range. Later an obvious paradoxical rise with intravenous glucose load. Glucagon in upper range of normal, falling with intravenous glucose

Summary

In this group the basal blood sugar level at 156 mg% is obviously lower than in the decerebrate cases, while the greatly raised cortisol and the normal HGH level are no different. The latter shows a delayed rise after 20 to 60 minutes. On the contrary the basal insulin level is low normal and there is only a very slight biphasic rise insecretion with intravenous glucose. Glucagon lies in the upper range of normal and shows a physiological fall with glucose.

Unconscious patients with acute midbrain syndrome and those with an acute mesencephalo-ponto-bulbar lesion are thus distinguished by the significant difference in the absolute concentration of the various substances concerned in glucose metabolism and in the kinetics of the changes in concentration after an intravenous glucose "load".

4.4.11. Unconscious Patients, Regardless of the Site and Level of the Lesion, or the Cerebral Cause

If we ignore the level of the lesion in the brain stem and if the unconsciousness is the sole criterion of this group, than the following situation is seen:

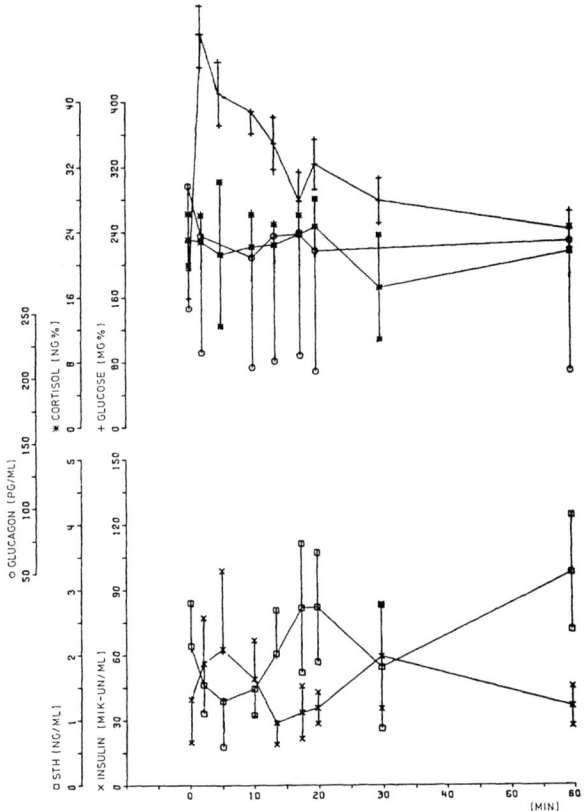

Fig. 73. Hyperglycaemia at 195 mg⁰/o, high cortisol at 23 ng⁰/o falling slightly with glucose. Basal insulin level high at 40 µU/ml. With intravenous glucose only a slight rise of insulin to 60 µU/ml. HGH drops and after 20 minutes shows only a slight rise above the initial value

The differences in concentration develop partly in a reciprocal manner. The excessive high values for glucagon in decerebration and the almost normal level in the patients with mesencephalo-ponto-bulbar syndrome give when combined definitely raised concentrations. The features of the differing kinetics are no longer apparent and the comparison to the total group of brain tumour patients on the first post-operative day shows only quantitative differences.

4.4.12. Unconscious Patients with the Clinical Signs of Brain Death

Individual Examples

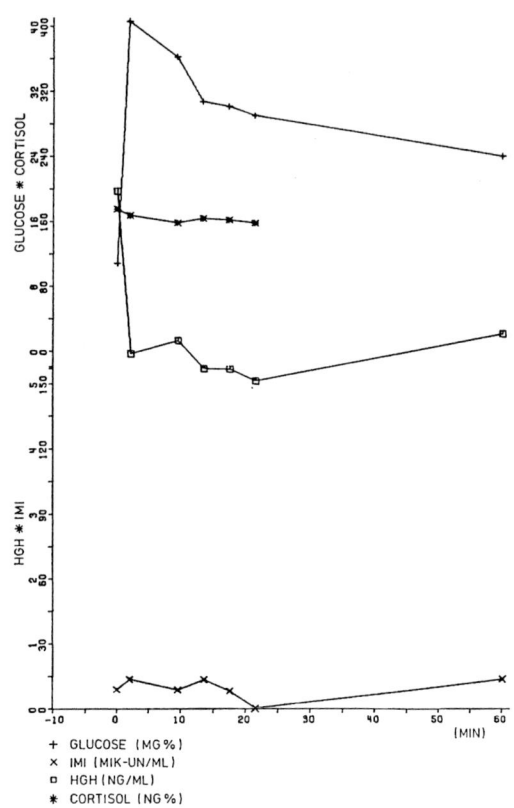

Fig. 74. Gunshot injury. 36-year-old man. Onset of brain death two hours before the test. Angiographic confirmation of intracranial circulatory arrest. Peripheral circulation, under artificial respiration N.A.D. Normothermia, renal excretion and blood gas values normal. Blood sugar normal. Cortisol level normal. Basal HGH raised, but with glucose a fall to a slightly raised normal value. Slight glucose-induced insulin secretion

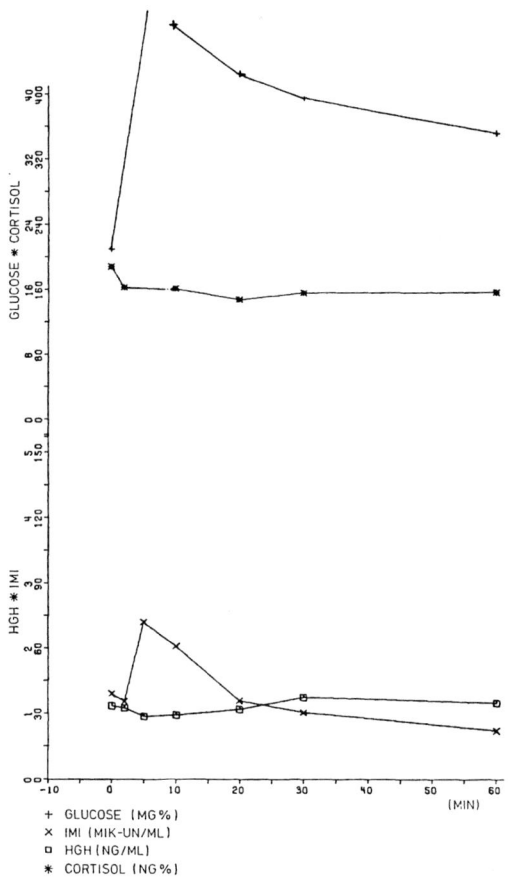

Fig. 75. Sixty-two-year-old man investigated 12 hours after onset of brain death, following a gunshot wound of brain. Hypothermia 31.8° (rectal). Raised blood sugar—210 mg⁰/o, normal to slightly raised values for HGH and cortisol, which showed a tendency to fall with glucose. Basal insulin raised and an obvious rise in secretion with intravenous glucose

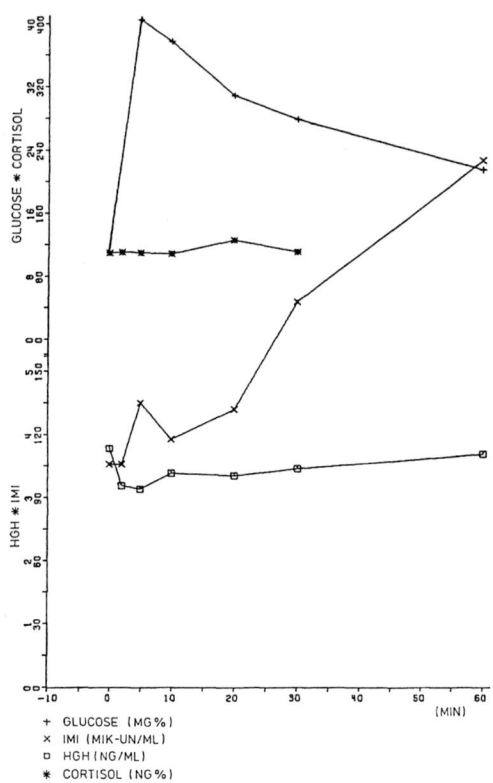

Fig. 76. Gunshot laceration of brain in a thirty-year-old man, investigated eleven
hours after onset of brain death. Normal blood sugar with marked increase of
basal insulin, a delayed but stronger induced insulin secretion. Cortisol in the
normal range. HGH slightly raised, slight fall with glucose

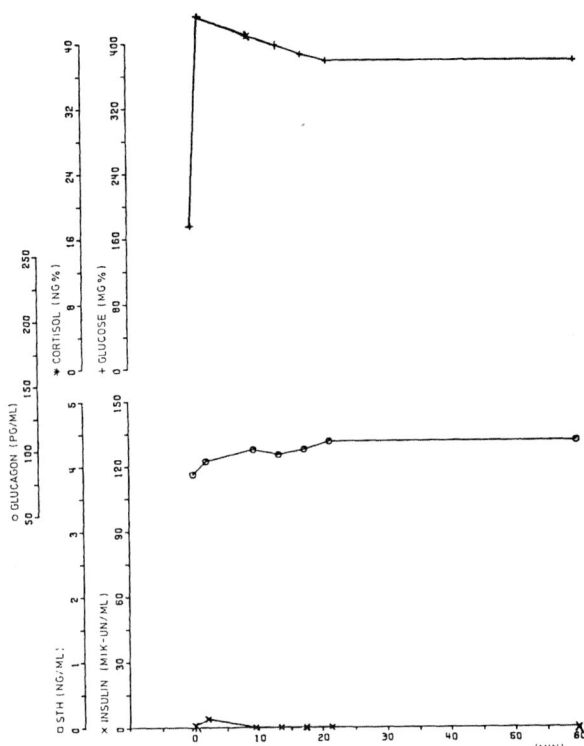

Fig. 77. Clinical brain death present for about 12 hours, condition having developed after severe closed craniocerebral injury and acute subdural haematoma. The core temperature was 32 °C, blood pressure was 70/50 mm Hg, urinary output 70 ml/hour. Moderate hyperglycaemia, absent or minimal basal and glucose-induced insulin secretion. Glucagon within normal limits without any significant change after glucose

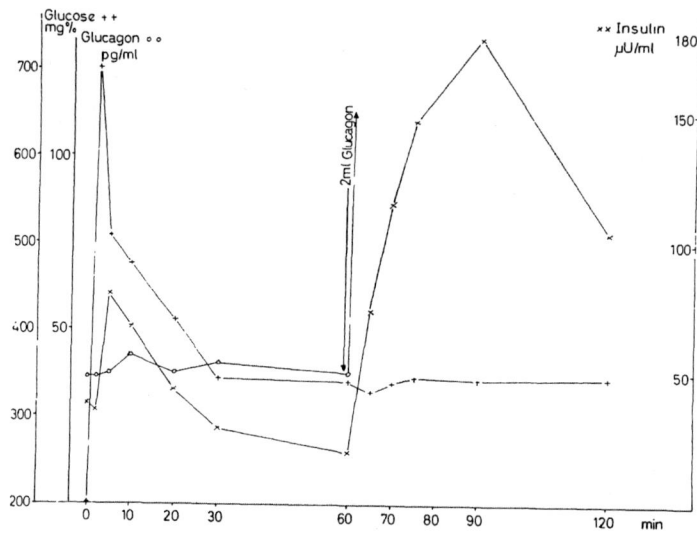

Fig. 78. Gunshot wound of brain. Investigation 12 hours after onset of brain death.
Core temperature 31.8 °C (rectal). Blood sugar 210 mg%. Acidosis pH 7.35, with
blood pressure no longer recordable. Low glucagon level was not affected by
intravenous glucose, however there was still reactive insulin secretion. With
exogenous glucagon there was marked secretion of insulin. The exogenous glucagon
did not alter the blood sugar level

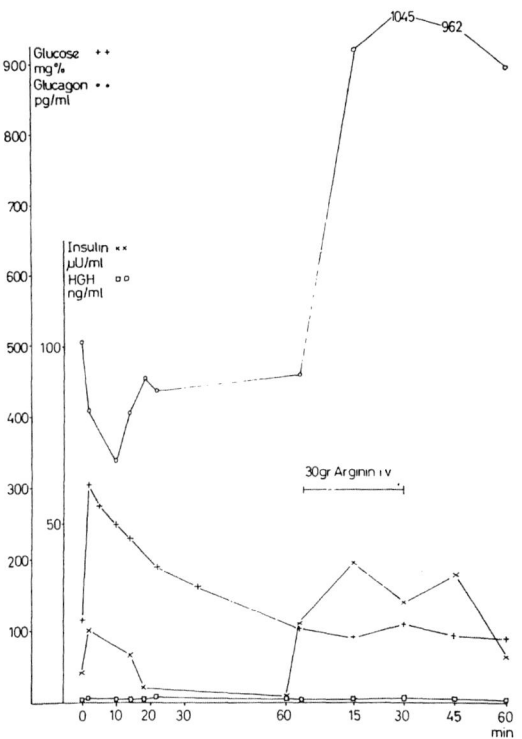

Fig. 79. Forty-five-year-old patient. Operation for a tentorial meningioma lying anterior to the pons and medulla oblongata. Comatose post-operatively. Diabetes insipidus. Raised blood sugar of 300 to 400 mg%. Hypothermia 35° (rectal). Onset of clinical brain death 30 hours after the operation and investigation 24 hours later. Peripheral blood pressure not recordable. Metabolic acidosis. Blood sugar 120 mg%. Basal insulin 10 µU/ml. Slight rise in secretion with i.v. glucose. Basal glucagon 505 pg/ml—brief drop with glucose. With an infusion of arginine further excessive glucagon secretion, marked output of insulin, but no stimulation of HGH

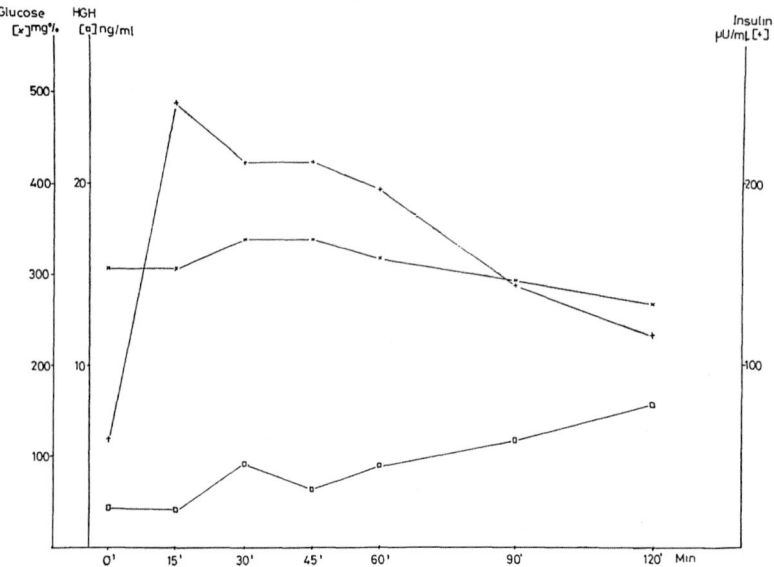

Fig. 80. Severe closed craniocerebral injury, cerebral coma, soon afterwards mid-brain decerebration and transition to stage of central death. Investigation 12 hours after the onset of brain death. Urinary output—N.A.D. Raised blood sugar 210 mg⁰/o. High insulin level at 60 μU/ml with arginine (0.5 kilo body weight in 30 minutes) a very marked rise to over 200 μU/ml, without the blood sugar being influenced by it in any way. However, a definite but delayed HGH secretion stimulated by arginine from a basal 2 ng/ml to 8 ng/ml after 120 minutes

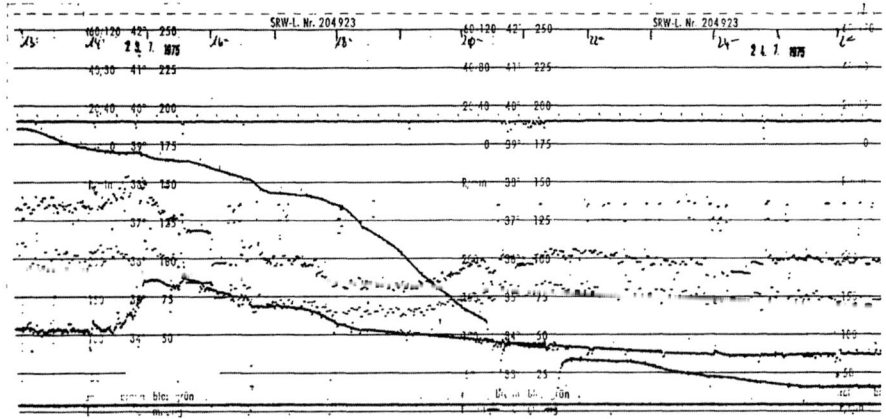

Fig. 81. Tracing of autonomic data from this patient. On the left hand side is the onset of brain death. Fall in blood pressure from 140/100 to 80/60 mm Hg (dots). Fall in temperature (upper continuous line). Fall in pulse rate after previously occurring rise, respiratory arrest had already occurred before this. On the right hand side of the tracing is the stage of brain death: cessation of respiration, hypothermia 32.5 (rectal), bradycardia 35/min without modulation of the pulse rate, blood pressure 100/75 mm Hg with slight support from i.v. fluids

Summary

The investigation of the glucose metabolism in these patients took place at varying times after the onset of brain death. The diagnosis and subsequent progress were different, while the state of the circulation and extent of the hypothermia also varied.

What is common to all, with the exception of Case 7, is the normal or slightly raised blood sugar, after hyperglycaemia before brain death.

Although all patients show the same clinical criteria of brain death, the behaviour of the individual "parameters" is quite variable: raised or normal HGH values which fell with glucose (patients 1–3) and rose with arginine infusion (patient 7), low HGH values under glucose load and absence of secretion with arginine (patient 6). Cortisol values were within the normal range (patients 1–3), basal insulin values with only moderate glucose-induced secretion (patients 1, 2, 4, and 6). On the other hand some patients (3.5) showed a high basal insulin and continuously stimulated insulin secretion (patient 5). Glucagon concentration may be low (patients 4 and 5) or markedly raised (patient 6).

4.4.13. Patients with Complete Lesions of the Upper Cervical Cord

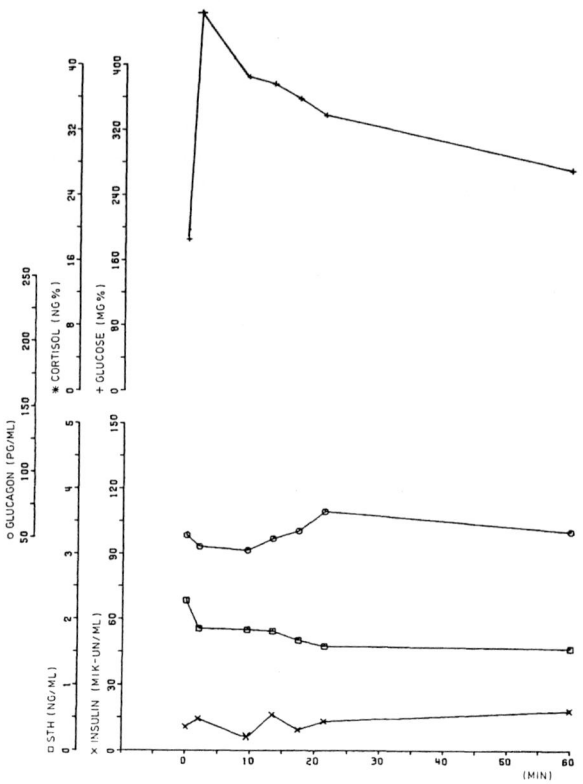

Fig. 82. Twenty-year-old man, fracture dislocation of C 4, almost the depth of
the vertebral body, fully conscious, complete flaccid motor and sensory tetraplegia
including the respiratory muscles. Rectal temperature 35.3°, bradycardia 60/min.
Investigated four days after the injury; moderately raised blood sugar at 180 mg%,
normal basal and very slight reactive insulin secretion. The glucagon is very low
(lowest mean value in the entire series) but it showed a slight tendency to fall with
glucose. HGH normal and normal fall with glucose

4.5. Mean Hourly Concentrations in the Various Groups, in Response to a Glucose Load

The representation of the mean concentration of the various substances per unit of time includes the basal as well as the reactive concentration and hence refers to the "decreasing quotient" or rate of disappearance of a substance. This facilitates a direct comparison in the various groups; while single estimations represent the momentary state, the calculation of the hourly mean concentration yields a figure for the effective concentration per unit of time. In this way inferences can be drawn about this complex regulation system. The individual mean hourly concentrations (HK/hour) were calculated by means of the trapezoidal rule. From this the mean value in the various groups was obtained and displayed with the confidence interval.

4.5.1. Glucose

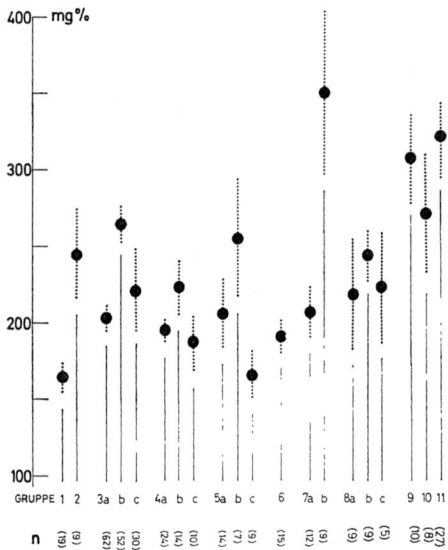

Fig. 83. Healthy subjects (*1*) show the lowest mean concentration of all groups. From the small confidence interval, conclusions can be drawn for a small scatter among the test subjects. They differ significantly from the diabetics (*2*). The entire group of intracranial space-occupying lesions (*3 a*) is in its turn significantly different from both of these. Their mean concentration is, by a small confidence interval, definitely higher than in the healthy. On the first post-operative day (*3 b*) there is a significant rise in the mean blood sugar concentration, which at this time is actually higher than in the diabetics. On the 7th post-operative day (*3 c*) the mean concentration falls, although the initial value has still not been reached. A significantly higher mean blood sugar concentration is found pre-operatively in the endocrine inactive pituitary tumours, than in the entire group of the intracranial space-occupying lesions. Also in this group there is a statistically confirmed rise of the mean concentration on the first post-operative day (*4 b*). On the 7th post-operative day (*4 c*) the mean concentration lies below the pre-operative value. Similar relationships exist with the endocrine active pituitary tumours. The pre-operative mean concentration (*5 a*) is significantly raised compared with the healthy controls: post-operatively (*5 b*) there is a definite rise of the mean blood sugar level. On the 7th post-operative day, in comparison to that it falls significantly below the pre-operative value and in the normal range for healthy subjects. The pre-operative mean value for the blood sugar in patients with anterior pituitary failure (*6*) is lower than in all other pre-operative groups, but statistically it is significantly higher than in the healthy controls. Cerebral tumours with involvement of the hypothalamus show no definite difference pre-operatively (*7 a*) in the mean blood sugar concentration, as compared with the other pre-operative groups. In this group it is also higher than in the healthy controls. Post-operatively (*7 b*) the mean blood sugar level is markedly raised and is found to be higher than in all the other post-operative groups, and also differs significantly from them. Superficial cortical cerebral hemisphere tumours show preoperatively

Summary

The mean blood-sugar concentration per hour after intravenous glucose load shows significant differences in the various groups.

The cerebral tumours show in general (3 a) and in their individual groups (4 a, 5 a, 7 a, 8 a) a statistically confirmed higher blood-sugar concentration than the healthy controls.

In all groups (b) compared with the pre-operative state (a) the trauma of operation leads to a further rise in the mean blood-sugar concentration which, even in the patients with cerebral hemisphere tumours (8) is also statistically significant. In these the rise of the mean blood sugar is less marked, but on the other hand it is most marked in the patients with para-hypothalamic tumours.

On the 7th day post-operatively (c) the mean blood-sugar level in the whole group of intracranial tumours had dropped, but it had still not reached the pre-operative level. On the other hand in the endocrine inactive (4 c) pituitary tumours and those with over-production of HGH (5 c) the mean blood-sugar concentration had dropped below the initial value. For the reasons already explained it was not possible to form a group 7 c. Two individual patients on the 7th post-operative day showed mean blood-sugar concentrations of 200 and 265 mg% respectively and also showed a fall almost to the pre-operative values. A third showed a very marked rise in the mean concentration to 758 mg%.

Patients with an acute midbrain syndrome (9) showed very high mean hourly blood-sugar concentrations. With the exception of the para-hypothalamic tumours the values were significantly higher than in all the post-operative groups on the first day.

Patients with acute mesencephalo-ponto-bulbar lesions (10) likewise showed a higher mean hourly blood-sugar concentration. It was lower than in the decerebrate cases and the entire group of those unconscious from a primarily cerebral cause.

(8 a) a definitely higher mean blood sugar level than the healthy controls. Post-operatively (8 a) it shows a slight rise. On the 7th post-operative day (8 c) the mean concentration returns again to the initial pre-operative value. Patients with acute midbrain syndrome (9), about 24 hours after the appearance of the neurological picture, show a marked rise in the mean blood-sugar level, which is significantly greater than in those post-operative groups which are free of complications. Only patients with cerebral tumours and involvement of the hypothalamus show a higher blood-sugar value. The acute mesencephalo-ponto-bulbar lesions also produce a definite rise in the mean blood sugar concentration, but it is less markedly raised than in the decerebrate cases. The entire group who are unconscious from a primarily cerebral cause (11) also show a marked increase in the mean blood-sugar level

4.5.2. Insulin

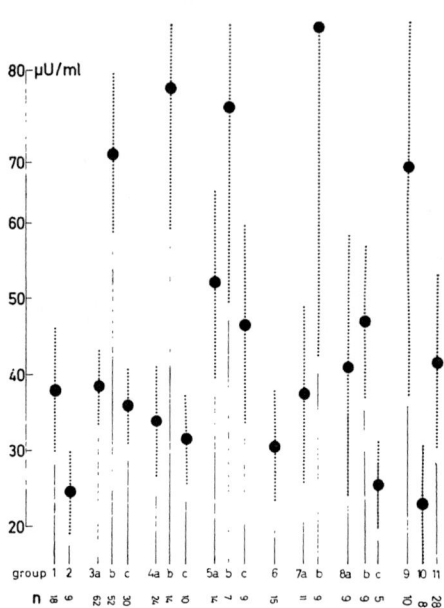

Fig. 84. The diagram of the mean hourly concentration of insulin with an intra-venous glucose load, shows significant differences between healthy (*1*) and dia-betics (*2*). Pre-operatively in the whole group of intracranial tumours (*3 a*) the insulin level is the same as in the healthy controls. Broken down into individual groups patients with para-hypothalamic tumours and, even more clearly, those with massive pituitary tumours show lower values than the whole group of cerebral tumours and the healthy. The lowest pre-operative values were recorded in patients with anterior pituitary insufficiency (*6*). Cerebral hemisphere tumours (*8 a*) shows some higher pre-operative values than the total group and the healthy. In the acromegalics the pre-operative values are very definitely raised. In the total group the trauma of operation leads to a marked increase in the mean insulin level in the different groups, which was moderate in the hemisphere tumours (*8 b*), definite in the acromegalics (*5 b*), extreme in the inactive pituitary tumours (*4 b*) and excessive with a broad confidence interval in the para-hypothalamic tumours. By the 7th post-operative day (*c*) the mean insulin concentration has fallen, even below the pre-operative value, in the total group (*3 c*) as well as in the inactive pituitary tumours (*4 c*) and in the acromegalics (*5 c*). In the cerebral hemisphere tumours (*5 c*) it fell to a very low range, as was observed in diabetics. The change in the mean insulin concentration in the individual groups between pre- and post-operative is also statistically significant. Only in the cerebral hemisphere tumours is the difference between the pre-operative and post-operative levels not statistically proven. The decerebrate (*9*) with a large confidence interval show high mean insulin concentrations. These are in the same range as the post-operative groups. In striking, statistically proven contrast to these are the very low values for patients with acute mesencephalo-ponto-bulbar lesions (*10*). They are lower than in any other groups. If the levels of the lesion in the brain stem are disregarded

Summary

The mean hourly concentration of insulin with an intravenous glucose load is pre-operatively as high as in the whole group of intracranial tumours as in the healthy, it is slightly lower in the para-hypothalamic tumours, definitely reduced in the inactive pituitary tumours and the lowest values are recorded in anterior pituitary insufficiency. Cerebral hemisphere tumours show slightly raised and acromegalics significantly higher values than in healthy.

Operation produced on the first day, in all groups, a raised insulin level in the blood, the lowest in hemisphere tumours and the most marked in para-hypothalamic tumours. By the seventh post-operative day the mean concentrations in all groups falls below the initial pre-operative values. Individual values of the mean concentration on the seventh day post-operatively in the para-hypothalamic tumours were: 29, 26, and 41 µU/ml.

The entire group of unconscious from cerebral causes (11) are not basically different from the healthy and the whole group of intra-cranial tumours.

If the levels of the lesion in the brain stem are taken into consideration there is a marked increase in the mean insulin level in the decerebrate, and extremely low values in patients with a mes-encephalo-ponto-bulbar syndrome (10).

---

and if unconsciousness from a cerebral cause is taken as the sole criterion the striking differences cancel each other out to some extent so that the mean insulin concentration in the unconscious (*11*) apparently is not changed as compared with the total group of intracranial tumours and the healthy

4.5.3. *Human Growth Hormone (HGH)*

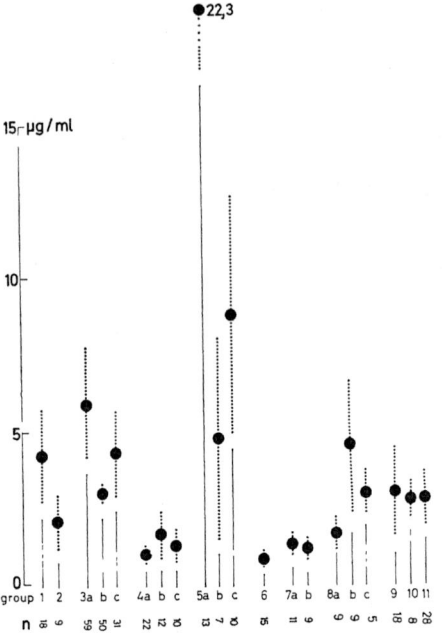

Fig. 85. The mean hourly concentration in ng/ml with an intravenous glucose load shows a significant difference between the healthy (*1*) and the diabetics (*2*). Also, hemisphere tumours pre-operatively (*8 a*) have a statistically verified lower value than the healthy. As might be expected the lowest concentrations are shown by the para-hypothalamic tumours (*7 a*), inactive pituitary tumours (*4 a*) and patients with anterior pituitary insufficiency (this group under 1 ng/ml). The confidence interval in these groups is very small. In the whole group of the intracranial tumours (*3 a*) including the acromegalics, the HGH is higher than in the healthy. Pituitary tumours with over-production of HGH (*5 a*) show high HGH concentrations. On the first day after operation on hormone-producing adenomas the HGH in the group 5 b shows a definite drop, as might be expected. In the whole group of intracranial tumours (*3 b*) there is an apparent fall of the HGH. The other groups however show a rise of HGH on the first post-operative day; this is most marked in the hemisphere tumours and is statistically significant, it is less in the inactive pituitary tumours and the mean concentration falls slightly in the para-hypothalamic tumours. On the seventh post-operative day the HGH drops in hemisphere tumours and in inactive pituitary tumours, however it does not reach the initial pre-operative values. On the other hand, acromegalics show a renewed overproduction of HGH, the concentration being twice as high as in the healthy, although still under 10 ng/ml. The entire group (*3 c*) likewise shows a rise of HGH on the seventh post-operative day as might be expected. Those unconscious from cerebral causes showed lower concentrations than the healthy and the HGH secretion is also definitely lower than in the hemisphere tumours on the first post-operative day. Patients with an acute midbrain syndrome (*9*) and those with acute mesencephalo-ponto-bulbar syndrome (*10*) show no difference from the total group of those unconscious from cerebral causes

Summary

Healthy subjects and diabetics show significant differences in the mean hourly HGH concentrations. The lowest values were recorded in patients with anterior pituitary insufficiency. The actual operation leads to a rise of HGH, which is marked and statistically significant in the hemisphere tumours and is less marked in the inactive pituitary tumours. The operative treatment of the HGH producing adenomas leads to a definite drop in acromegalics and, naturally, in the whole group of intracranial tumours.

On the seventh post-operative day the HGH concentrations fall in cerebral hemisphere and inactive pituitary tumours, but they do not reach the initial pre-operative values. On the other hand a fresh rise of the mean HGH concentration can be shown in the acromegalics and the whole group of intracranial tumours.

The unconscious shown lower concentrations than the healthy or the operated hemisphere tumours. The levels of the lesion in the brain stem (9, 10) have no significant influence on the total hourly HGH secretion.

4.5.4. Cortisol

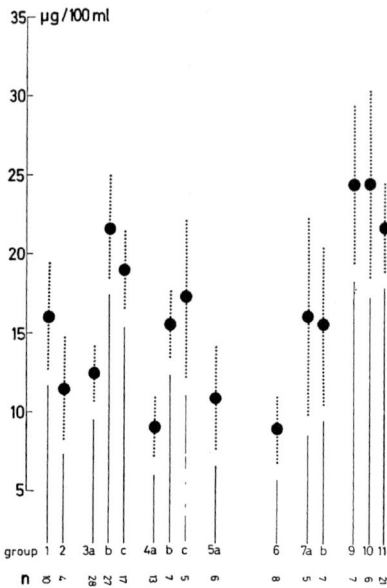

Fig. 86. The mean hourly cortisol concentration under an intravenous glucose load shows definitely lower values in diabetics (2) at 12 ng% , than in the healthy (1) at 16 ng%. The whole group of intracranial space-occupying lesions likewise shows lower concentrations pre-operatively (3 a) compared with the healthy. As might be expected they are still lower, at 8 ng% in patients with in-active pituitary tumours. It is lowest in the group of patients with anterior pituitary insufficiency and it is likewise reduced in the acromegalics pre-opera-tively (5 a). On the other hand, the para-hypothalamic tumours, show pre-operative concentrations similar to the healthy controls. Operation leads to a significant rise in the blood cortisol in the whole group (3 b) and in the inactive pituitary tumours (4 b) and this is still apparent on the seventh post-operative day. In the whole group it drops compared with the first post-operative day, but in the inactive pituitary tumours it rises still further. On the other hand the cortisol concentration does not change post-operatively in the para-hypothalamic tumours. There are only isolated observations on the hemisphere tumours and these also show a very marked rise of cortisol on the first post-operative day, which is falling again on the seventh post-operative day. The highest hourly cortisol con-centrations were found in the decerebrate (9) and in patients with mesencephalo-ponto-bulbar syndrome (10) and in the whole group of the unconscious (11). These three groups did not in any way differ from each other

Summary

Diabetics, pituitary tumours and the whole group of intracranial tumours pre-operatively show strikingly lower mean hourly cortisol concentration than the healthy. Smaller values were recorded in patients with anterior pituitary insufficiency. The operation leads on the first pre-operative day to a significant rise of cortisol which is falling again by the seventh post-operative day. The para-hypo-thalamic tumours have a normal cortisol level pre-operatively and there is no evidence of any rise of the level post-operatively.

Decerebrate cases and patients with the mesencephalo-ponto-bulbar syndrome show the highest mean hourly concentration of cortisol in all the groups. They differ minimally or not at all from the entire group of those unconscious from a cerebral cause.

4.5.5. Glucagon

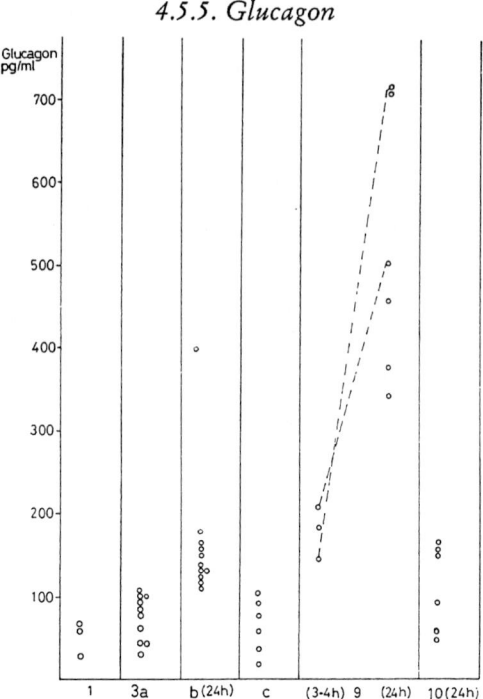

Fig. 87. On account of the small number of investigations, the mean hourly glucagon concentrations in response to an intravenous glucose load have not been averaged in several groups, but are shown is individual values. In the healthy (*1*) they are low at 30 to 60 pg/ml. Intracranial tumours pre-operatively (*3 a*) show mean concentrations in the normal range or slightly above, up to 100 pg/ml. The trauma of operation leads to a very definite rise in the mean hourly concentration of glucagon up to twice the initial values. On the seventh post-operative day they have again returned to the pre-operative values. In the decerebrate cases (*9*) one is able to recognize a relationship between the mean hourly glucagon concentration and the time of the brain stem lesion. Investigation one hour after the onset of injury show statistically raised values. These same patients when "stressed" with a glucose load about twenty-four hours after the onset of decerebration, show extreme values of 500 to 700 pg/ml. Five further patients with a decerebration syndrome when investigated 24 hours later, also showed maximally raised concentrations. In contrast to the acute midbrain syndrome, the concentrations recorded in the acute mesencephalo-ponto-bulbar syndrome were in the normal range or slightly above it. From the other groups there are isolated observations. A maximal rise of mean concentration to 399 pg/ml was seen on the first day after operation on an olfactory groove meningioma which was displacing the hypothalamus; the pre-operative values had been in the normal range. The concentrations in two patients with irreversible failure of cerebral function (brain death) were in the normal range. A patient with complete transection of the upper cervical cord showed a very low mean hourly glucagon concentration with a figure of 57 pg/ml. Two unconscious patients without verifiable levels of the brain stem lesion, showed mean concentrations of 248 and 285 respectively

Summary

Low mean hourly concentrations under intravenous glucose load are reported in the healthy, in patients with clinical signs of brain death and in a patient with complete transection of the upper cervical cord. Normal to slightly raised values are found pre-operatively in brain tumours. The trauma of operation leads to a rise of the mean glucagon concentration to twice the initial pre-operative values. These are reached once again by the seventh post-operative day.

Decerebrate cases a few hours after the brain-stem injury show a markedly increased mean glucagon concentration, which after twenty-four hours is extremely raised. In contrast to this group the mean concentration in patients with acute mesencephalo-ponto-bulbar syndrome is in the normal range or slightly above. Unconscious patients without any demonstrable lesion in the brain stem show higher concentrations than patients with brain tumours post-operatively.

4.5.6. Mean Concentrations of the Catecholamines in 24 Hour Urine

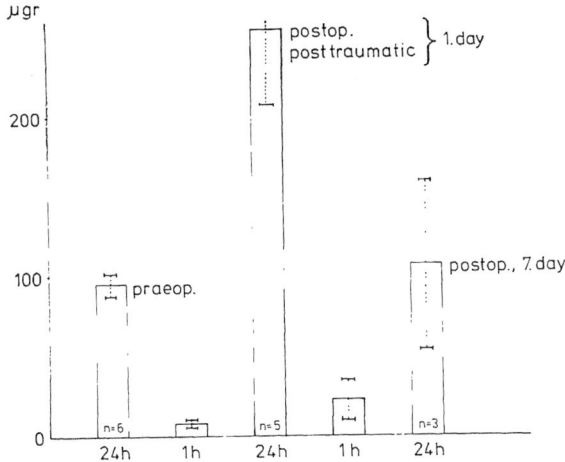

Fig. 88. The daily urinary output of catecholamines in certain brain tumours, was measured pre-operatively, on the first and seventh days post-operatively. While the pre-operative mean value was about 95 µg, it has risen by the first day post-operatively to over 200 µg. In a large series in 1973 Lorenz showed that the highest values are seen in severe closed craniocerebral injuries and that remarkable differences in output occur depending on the level of the lesion. Patients with diencephalic failure, and decerebrate cases show figure of 67 µg and 153 µg, respectively. On the seventh post-operative day the pre-operative values are almost reached once again

The lowest hourly and daily amounts excreted were recorded in a young man, on the first day after a complete transection of the upper cervical spinal cord, the result of a fracture dislocation. Whilst as a rule the excretion on the first day post-operatively lay between 10 and 25 µg per hour and for the 24 hours was over 200 µg, in the aforementioned patient values of under 2 µg per hour and of 40 µg in 24 hours were noted. In a further patient with an upper cervical cord lesion (C 3/4) a figure of 15 µg in 24 hours was recorded. Consequently the resting secretion or the basal output of catecholamines free of any CNS control appears to lie in this range. The catecholamines excreted in the urine consist essentially of adrenaline and noradrenaline secreted by the adrenal medulla. The amount of noradrenaline set free in the synaptic gap is registered only in tiny fractions or not at all by the measurement of the catecholamine excretion. Consequently it does not allow us to draw conclusions on the general activity of the sympathetic nervous system. Even the methods of estimating catecholamines in the blood involve a still larger margin of error and can only produce here a quantitative improvement, as a large proportion of the noradrenaline is reabsorbed locally and resynthesized in the synaptic gap and hence does not appear in the blood.

4.6. The Molar Insulin-Glucagon Quotient in the Various Groups

According to Unger (1972) the molar relationship of insulin to glucagon is calculated:

$$\frac{\text{Insulin } \mu U/ml}{\text{Glucagon } pg/ml} \times 23.3$$

However the basal value alone is not used for the calculation of these quotient, but the mean concentration for one hour under an intravenous glucose load, in order to obtain a parameter for the many-sided regulation of the basal and glucose-induced secretion of these hormones (Fig. 89).

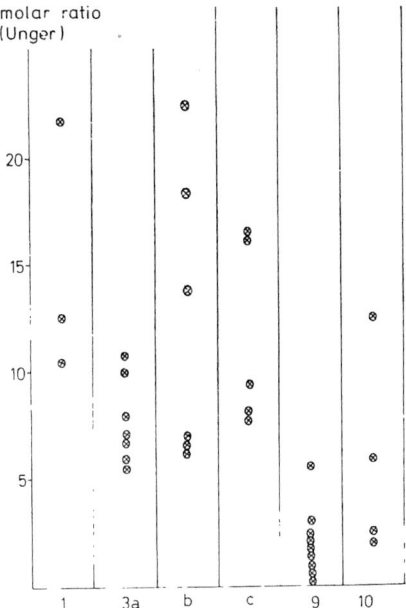

Fig. 89. In healthy subjects after previous feeding the quotient is over 10. In intra-cranial tumours pre-operatively (*3 a*) it is reduced to values between 5 and 10. On the first post-operative day it is either unchanged or slightly raised. Also on the seventh post-operative day there is still a tendency to rise, as compared with before the operation. Patients with a midbrain syndrome (*9*) on the contrary show a very marked fall, most values being between 0.2 and 2. Similarly in patients with a mesencephalo-ponto-bulbar syndrome most of the figures are low. Two patients with the clinical signs of brain death showed extremely low values of 0.1 to 0.2. In the patient with the high cervical transection the quotient was 5.7. On the first day after operation on an olfactory groove meningioma involving the hypo-thalamus the quotient was 7.2

Summary

The "molar ratio" regarded by Unger as a measure of anabolism and catabolism is lowered in brain tumours pre-operatively as compared with the healthy, *i.e.* it is shifted in the direction of catabo-lism. The actual operation leads to a slight rise of the quotient, which is still apparent even on the seventh post-operative day.

In contrast the decerebrate cases show a markedly lowered quoti-ent and in these patients the metabolism shows a marked trend to-wards catabolism. In patients with mesencephalo-ponto-bulbar lesion there is a greater fluctuation of the quotient but on the whole it is also reduced in this group.

4.7. Pharmacokinetic Investigation of the Concentration Pattern and of the Assimilation of the Blood Glucose After an Intravenous Glucose Load

The constant K 2 as a measure of the glucose assimilation, and the transfer as a dimension of the turnover of glucose were obtained separately for each individual investigation and plotted for the individual groups as mean and confidence interval, after the necessary mathematical correction when there had been urinary excretion of glucose.

4.7.1. Glucose Assimilation

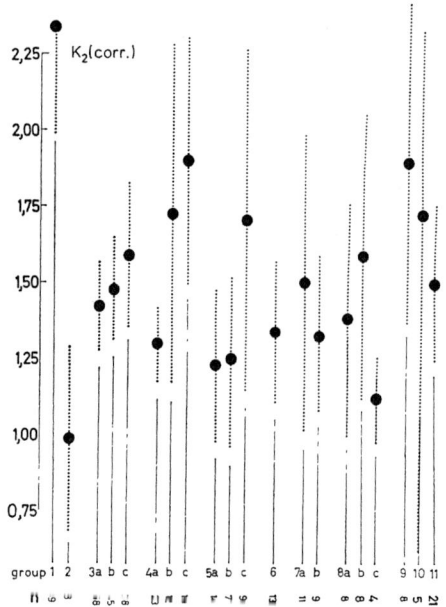

Fig. 90. All brain tumours showed pre-operatively (*3 a*) a reduction in glucose assimilation compared with healthy subjects (*1*). A similarly statistically significant difference distinguished them from the diabetics (*2*). When considered in their individual groups the hemisphere tumours (*8 a*) have a slightly lower, and para-hypothalamic tumors a slightly raised K 2, as compared with the entire group. The assimilation is definitely reduced in the non-active pituitary tumours (*4*). K 2 is smallest in the group of acromegalics (*5 a*) which might be expected as a proportion of these patients is diabetic. With tumours involving the hypothalamus (*7 b*) the trauma of operation leads on the first post-operative day to a slight drop, but in all the other groups to an increase, in the assimilation. This is small in the acromegalics (*5 b*) and the whole group of all intracranial tumours (*3 b*), definite in the hemisphere tumours (*8 b*) and greatest in the inactive pituitary tumours (*4 b*).

Summary

The assimilation constant K 2 shows a statistically significant difference between the healthy and diabetics. The group of all the intracranial tumours showed, in comparison with the healthy, a statistically confirmed lower, and in comparison with the diabetics a higher assimilation. Also the individual groups of brain tumours show a significantly lower K 2 than the healthy.

With the exception of the para-hypothalamic tumours—where there is a slight drop in K 2—in all groups operation leads to a rise of assimilation on the first post-operative day, smallest in the HGH-producing tumours and most obvious in the inactive pituitary tumours. On the seventh post-operative day the pituitary tumours experience a further rise of the K 2 value, but in the hemisphere tumours it falls definitely below the pre-operative value.

The decerebrate showed the highest assimilation of glucose as compared with all other groups on the first post-operative day. It is greater than in the entire group of the unconscious.

Patients with acute mesencephalo-ponto-bulbar syndrome and those with clinical signs of brain death do not behave in a uniform manner.

On the seventh post-operative day in the total group (*3 c*), in the inactive (*4 c*) and active (*5 c*) pituitary tumours, there is a further increase in assimilation, which is most marked in the acromegalics, while hemisphere tumours show a distinct drop in glucose assimilation on the seventh post-operative day. Individual patients with para-hypothalamic tumours show values of 1.32 and 0.88. The decerebrate group (*9*) shows on the first day the highest assimilation for glucose of all the post-operative groups. The greatest scatter for K 2 is found in patients with mesencephalo-ponto-bulbar lesions (*10*). As regards glucose assimilation, these do not form a uniform group. All the unconscious (*11*) show a distinctly lower K 2 than the decerebrate. Patients with the clinical signs of brain death behave in a variable manner. As regards the size of the mean insulin concentration those with a low secretion (Fig. 74 and 77) show a very low K 2 of 0.46 or 0.74, while those with an adequate production of insulin (Fig. 75 and 76) show an elimination-constant of 1.49 to 1.77. The patient with a complete high cervical cord lesion and almost absent insulin secretion, had an extremely small K 2 of 0.69

4.7.2. Glucose Transfer

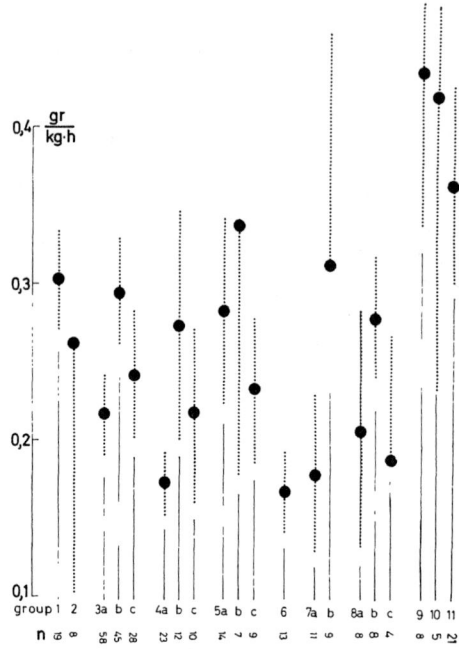

Fig. 91. The figure designated as "transfer" which is calculated from the behaviour of the glucose concentration after a glucose load gives a measure of the absolute amount of glucose per kilogram body weight and per hour, which is transferred in flux equilibrium, *i.e.*, with a constant blood sugar level. With a small confidence interval the transfer in the healthy controls (*1*) is 0.3 g/kg/hour; the group of all the diabetics (*2*) shows marked fluctuations of their glucose transfer. All patients with brain tumours have pre-operatively (*3 a*) a smaller turnover of glucose than the healthy. This difference is small in the acromegalics (*5 a*), well marked and statistically significant in the group of all brain tumours (*3 a*) and raised and statistically confirmed in patients with inactive pituitary tumours (*4 a*) and in para-hypothalamic tumours (*7 a*). Those patients with clinical and endocrinological criteria of anterior pituitary insufficiency actually show the smallest glucose consumption. Hemisphere tumours show a large scatter within the group. The mean is definitely below that of the healthy controls. The trauma of the operation leads, in all groups, to an increase in the utilisation of glucose, definite but without statistical confirmation in acromegalics (*5 b*), and hemisphere tumours (*8 b*), marked and statistically confirmed in the total group of all brain tumours (*3 b*) in the inactive pituitary tumours (*4 b*) and the para-hypothalamic tumours (*7 b*). The latter and the acromegalics on the first post-operative day actually reach the same transfer value as the healthy. On the seventh post-operative day the utilisation of glucose drops in all groups, but in the whole group (*3 c*), as in the inactive pituitary tumours (*4 c*), it is still higher than the pre-operative control value. In the acromegalics (*5 c*), the hemisphere tumours (*8 c*), and the para-hypothalamic tumours (individual values 0.154 and 0.179 respectively), it is still below this

Summary

The glucose transfer in g/kg/hour with a marked scatter in the individual groups shows a striking difference between the healthy and those patients with brain tumour. In acromegaly the drop in the transfer is small, it is marked and statistically significant in the group of all brain tumours, in the inactive pituitary tumours and the para-hypothalamic tumours. Even patients with cerebral hemisphere tumours also have a reduced glucose transfer pre-operatively. The lowest transfer value of all groups was recorded in the patients with anterior pituitary insufficiency.

One day after the operation there is a rise in the utilization of glucose, less in hemisphere tumours and acromegalics, marked and statistically significant in the whole group, in inactive pituitary tumours and the para-hypothalamic tumours. On the seventh post-operative day the transfer falls in all groups, but it does not reach the pre-operative values in the total group or in the inactive pituitary tumours. It falls short of this in the acromegalics, hemisphere tumours and para-hypothalamic tumours.

Compared with healthy subjects the decerebrate have a statistically significantly raised utilization, the extent of which is not attained by any of the post-operative groups. The unconscious likewise show a raised utilization, but this is less than in the patients with an acute midbrain syndrome. Patients with irreversible central loss of function (brain death) utilize extremely low or subnormal amounts of glucose, in relation to their insulin secretion.

---

on the seventh post-operative day. The decerebrate (9) show a marked, statistical verified rise in the glucose utilisation as compared with the healthy, and this was found to be higher than in all the post-operative groups. Also patients with mesencephalo-ponto-bulbar brain-stem lesions (10) show a similar transfer with, actually, a marked scatter within the group. Those unconscious from a cerebral cause show a raised glucose utilisation, which is still lower than in the decerebrate. Patients with irreversible central loss of function (brain death) show, in analogy with the low K 2 and mean insulin value (Fig. 44 and 47) an extremely low utilisation of 0.076 and a very small "transfer" of 0.154 g/kg-hour. With more obviously normal insulin secretion and normal K 2 values (Fig. 75 and 76) values of 0.3 and 0.191 g/kg-hour respectively were obtained

4.8. Inhibition Tests with Somatostatin

In some cases inhibition test with somatostatin were done (250 mcg as a bolus, 750 mcg as infusion for 60 minutes).

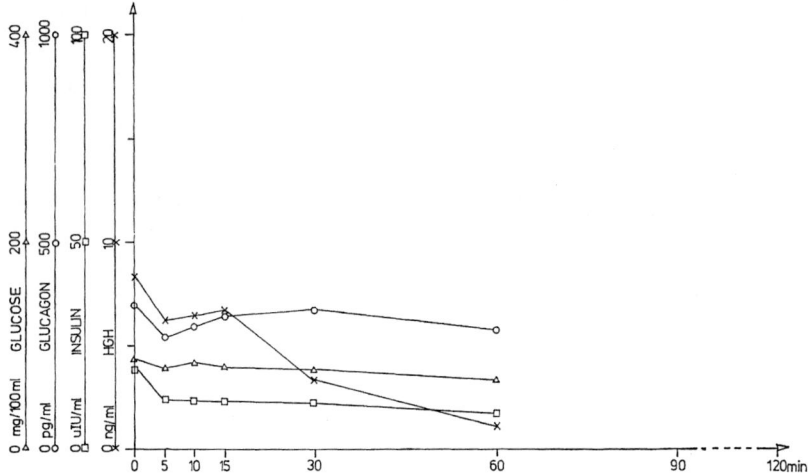

Fig. 92. Healthy fasting subject after somatostatin bolus and infusion: basal values of glucose (85 mg%), insulin (18 uIU/ml), glucagon (320 pg/ml) and HGH (8.5 ng/ml) are falling through 60 minutes, there is a rebound phenomenon of glucagon after 10 minutes

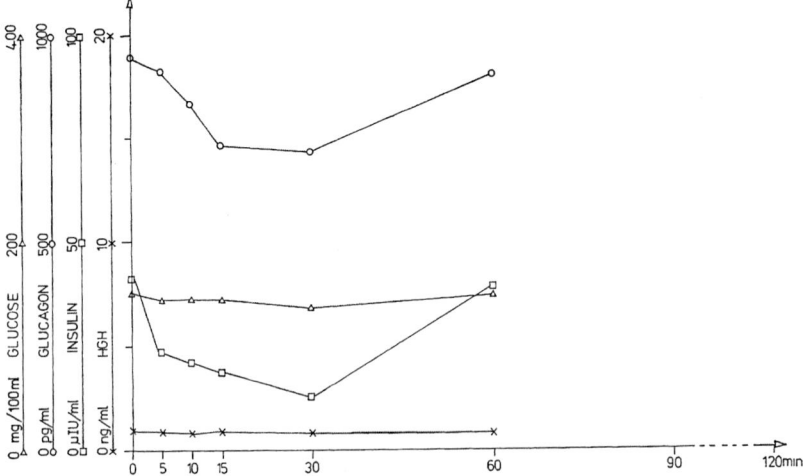

Fig. 93. Clinical syndrome of midbrain-herniation due to spontaneous occipito-parietal haematoma: moderate basal hyperglycaemia at 180 mg%, largely increased basal insulin and extremely raised glucagon levels. On somatostatin, very marked drop of insulin and glucagon, but after 60 minutes inspite of continuous infusion of somatostatin initial values are reached again. Glucose level and very low HGH unchanged

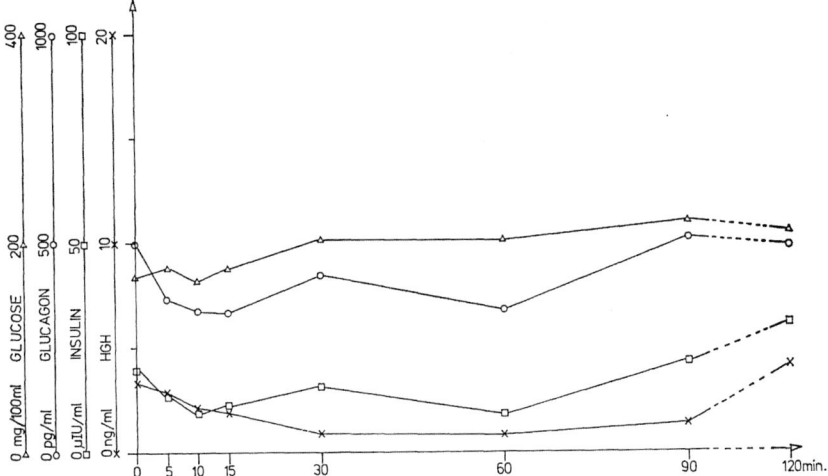

Fig. 94. A 24-years old youth since 3 days in midbrain herniation because of too late discovered and then operated epidural haematoma: Moderate basal hyperglycaemia of 180 mg⁰/o and increased basal values for insulin (20 uIU/ml) and glucagon (500 pg/ml). These hormones are well lowered by somatostatin, but reach almost initial levels after 60 minutes. Glucose stays unchanged, hormonal basal HGH level is lowered

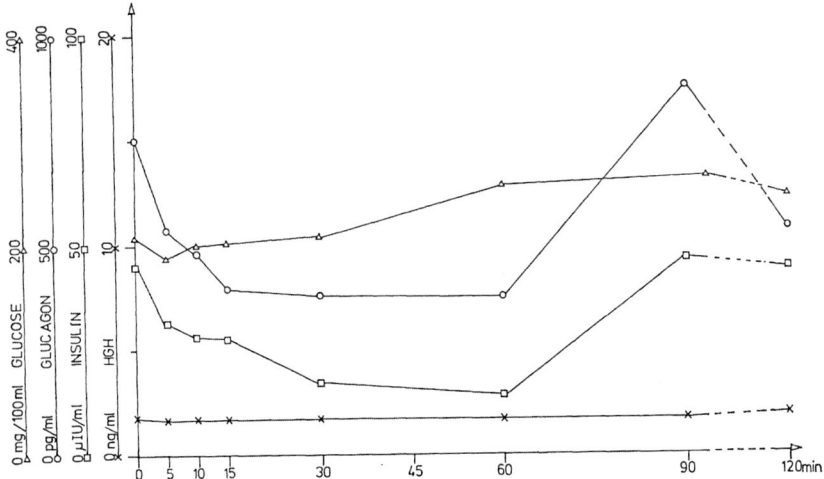

Fig. 95. Mesencephalo-bulbar-coma 3 days after bilateral anterior cerebral infarction after clipping of an a.c.a. aneurysm: moderate hyperglycaemia of 204 mg⁰/o, strong elevation of basal insulin (45 uIU/ml) and glucagon levels (750 pg/ml). Hormones are dramatically lowered throughout infusion time and rise again after discontinuing. In contrast, basal HGH stays unchanged and glucose level slightly increases

9*

Summary

Whereas in healthy subjects somatostatin leads to lowered levels of HGH, insulin, glucagon and glucose, in midbrain syndrome glucagon and insulin are suppressed only temporarily and rise again in spite of continuous infusion, glucose level is not changing. In case of fading sympathetic activity as in mesencephalobulbar damage, insulin and glucagon are markedly inhibited throughout the administration of the drug, they rise again after discontinuing.

5. Consideration of the Results and Discussion

Disturbances of blood sugar homeostasis after various general surgical operations have been reported by Schultis (1971), Howard (1955), McNamara, Molot, Stremple, and Sleeman (1971), Ross, Johnston, Welborne, and Wright (1966), and Stremmel (1972, 1974). Hyperglycaemia and also glycosuria were observed and appeared to be related to the severity of the operation or of the injury. The disturbance in the utilization of glucose, which is measurable by a reduction of the K value has been discussed as one of the causes of hyperglycaemia, increased utilization of free fatty acids is supposed to be another one. An increased secretion of anti-insulin hormones is suggested as a further cause. The inhibition of glucose-induced insulin secretion during operation (Allison, Tomlin, and Chamberlain 1969, Stremmel 1972), after burns (Hinton, Allison, Littlejohn, and Lloyd 1971), or after myocardial infarction (Allison, Prowse, and Chamberlain 1967) is regarded as an additional cause for the hyperglycaemia which is seen. In the above-mentioned situations of stress, the increased secretion of catecholamines is accepted as a common aetiological factor. Stremmel (1972) has been able to abolish the inhibition of secretion by the administration of alpha-receptor blockers and he also managed to break through this inhibition by the simultaneous administration of arginine (Stremmel, Kummerle, Kruse-Jarres 1975). An increase in the basal and glucose-induced insulin level has been described a few hours to a day after operations (Geser, Schultis, and Diedrichson 1970, Stremmel 1970, 1972, Allison, Hinton, and Chamberlain 1968). It was explained by a post-operative insulin resistance (Geser 1974, Allison, Hinton, and Chamberlain 1968), as the glucose assimilation is diminished for a few hours after any operations. Stremmel (1972) on the other hand, explained the surplus insulin secretion by the continuing production of insulin in the beta-cells during the intra-operative inhibition. Also in animal experiments, hyperglycaemia and hyperinsulinaemia have been observed after operation and trauma (Koch 1974).

Metabolic disturbances such as hyperglycaemia were described by Gissel in 1933 after brain trauma although they only appeared in patients with disturbances of consciousness. Oberdisse and Rauser (1949) and Oberdisse (1950) had found "inverse" patterns in acute brain injuries after an insulin load, *i.e.* the blood sugar only falls very little or not at all, or it even rises. Extensive chronic lesions of the hypothalamus can show intact regulation of carbohydrate metabolism (Oberdisse 1951), whereas acute lesions can bring about diverse responses to stimulation. With hyperglycaemia after extirpation of pituitary tumours and after trauma there was a noticeable insulin resistance. This "inversion" was only observed with raised intracranial pressure or in the phase of oedema in the third and fourth days after operation.

Hyperglycaemia and insulin resistance were also observed after subarachnoid haemorrhage (Hallpike, Claveria, Cohen, and Lascelle 1971). King, Knowles, McLaurin, and Lewis (1971) have found hyperglycaemia and low insulin levels in brain injuries dependent on the duration of the loss of consciousness. Mouawad and van Laere (1973) and Keymolen-Jardin, Mouawad, Claeys-de Clerq, van Laere, Levin, and Borkowski (1973) had regarded the hyperglycaemia in cranio-cerebral injuries as the response to a complete hormonal disturbance. A paradoxical HGH rise in response to glucose had been noted as the only typical nervous element. Mouawad and van Laere (1974) reporting on 128 brain injuries were able to establish a correlation between hyperglycaemia and the severity of the trauma as well as the mortality. Blood sugar levels of over 500 mg^0/o were seen and they were interpreted as partly unspecific and produced by the stress, but for the most part as a result of the brain injury.

In addition the production of hormones antagonistic to insulin and the resultant reduced glucose utilization, as well as the partial or total inhibition of insulin secretion are considered as causes of the hyperglycaemia. This also poses a problem in treatment.

In contrast to the inhibition of glucose-induced insulin secretion encouragement of glucagon secretion is found in stress resulting from injuries and other acute situations. Clinical observations of a high blood glucagon level have been made in traumatic shock (Halmagyi 1969, Lindsay, Santeusanio, Braaten, Faloona, and Unger 1974), in burns (Wilmore, Lindsay, Moyland, Faloona, Pruitt, and Unger 1974), in severe infection (Bruder *et al.* 1973), in non-ketotic hyperosmolar coma (Lindsay *et al.* 1974) and after excessive physical exertion (Böttger, Schlein, Faloona, Knochel, and Unger 1972). These observations suggest that the common cause of the rise of glucagon in these acute conditions of stress lies in the neural or catecholamine-determined stimulation, because in all the cases specified there was never any hypoglycaemia which would lead to glucagon secretion, but the glucose concentration was, in fact, slightly raised.

Our own investigations regarding the disturbance of glucose metabolism in acute brain lesions confirm the influence of the central nervous system on the carbohydrate metabolism which has been noted by many earlier investigators. The disturbance of homeostasis consists always of an elevation of the blood sugar level; one never sees a hypoglycaemia produced by the central nervous system.

The slight post-operative hyperglycaemia which is described after general surgical procedures in the literature can also be confirmed after operations on intracranial space-occupying lesions. The mean concentration of glucose was still raised even on the seventh post-operative day. The mean concentration of glucose pre-operatively was already significantly higher than in the healthy. This corresponded to the lower K 2 value pre-operatively, in comparison with healthy subjects, while the mean insulin concentration pre-operatively corresponded to that of the healthy. The lowered K 2 and the raised mean values for blood sugar concentration which are observed pre-operatively in comparison with healthy subjects, probably have their cause in the repression of key enzymes for glycolysis, resulting from fasting, insufficient pre-operative feeding and reduced bodily activity (Malaisse, Sener, Levy 1975).

The high post-operative insulin levels which were found by previous investigators in general surgical material can be confirmed in the whole group of intracranial space-occupying lesions, as well as separately in the inactive and active pituitary tumours and the para-hypothalamic tumours. On the seventh post-operative day the insulin levels fall short of the pre-operative mean concentrations or have again reached it.

Clear correlations were established between the location of the cerebral lesion and/or the level of the lesion in the brainstem and the extent and pattern of the disturbances of carbohydrate metabolism.

The highest mean blood sugar levels were recorded on the first day after operation in tumours compressing or displacing the hypothalamus. These high sugar levels were connected with a synchronous elevation of the mean concentrations of insulin and glucagon, whereas HGH and cortical remained unchanged in the low normal range compared with pre-operatively.

The analysis of this rise in the blood sugar showed first of all that only a minor role is played by any peripheral disturbance of glucose utilization. The drop in the constant K 2 is only slight compared with the pre-operative value. Generally speaking it is only in this group that the assimilation of glucose as measured by the K 2 is lower in comparison with the pre-operative. In all other groups the K 2 was found post-operatively to be slightly raised in comparison with pre-operatively. In comparison with the group of healthy controls the glucose assimilation post-operatively was definitely lowered. The comparison within the various groups preoperatively and on the first and seventh post-operative days shows that the factor of the brain operation does not lower the glucose assimilation in muscle and fat cells, but leads to a slight increase in the peripheral utilization, which appears to be very marked in the group of non-active pituitary adenomas.

This slight fall in assimilation seen in the group of para-hypothalamic tumours cannot be the cause of the marked hyperglycaemia. This is explained much more by the increased production of glucose.

This again is a sequel to the increased central nervous stimulation. The consideration of the findings based on anatomy (Ban 1966) and neurophysiology (Oomura, Ono, Ooyama, and Wayner 1969) as well as our own results lead to the conclusion that the blood sugar concentration is monitored in the ventro-medial and lateral hypothalamus. When there is hypoglycaemia the neurohumoral secretion of HGH and ACTH results, while through the diencephalic nuclei of the sympathetic—the "area sympathica" of Ban—glycogenolysis is immediately stimulated in the liver cells through neural pathways, as well as glucagon secretion in the pancreas and catecholamine secretion in the adrenal medulla, while insulin secretion in the beta-cells is inhibited. On the other hand a rise of the blood sugar level leads to a drop in the HGH and ACTH (i.e. the cortisol) level, particularly with slightly raised values (Wilder 1931) and to a reduction in the output of adrenaline and noradrenaline from the adrenal medulla. The secretion of insulin is stimulated and that of glucagon inhibited. It is established that the islet cells of the pancreas also function independently of the nervous system and they regulate the secretion of their hormones according to the level of the blood sugar. Irritation and damage to the hypothalamus thus leads to a neuronal pattern of stimulation the same as when a hypoglycaemia were present. This behaviour suggests the existence of different mechanisms. The neuronal input and hence the "set point" (Schade 1970) has changed or the hypothalamic neurones are actually hypoglycaemic in spite of the raised blood glucose. In this connexion it is a significant fact in our experience that even extensive chronic displacements and destructive lesions of the hypothalamus from slowing growing tumours never cause a hyperglycaemia. On the contrary, on account of the defective or absent regulation of HGH and ACTH, patients show lower blood sugar levels and a hypersentivity to insulin. If such patients have now an operation on a tumour which has already damaged the hypothalamus, after a latent period of a few hours a marked and increasing hyperglycaemia appears. Some oedema of the brain is to be expected after such intervention in the region of the hypothalamus. If this leads to a disturbance of membrane transport for glucose it could lead hypothetically to intracellular glucopaenia. Even with normal or raised blood sugar levels this intra-cellular glucose depletion must lead to the neuronal and neurohumoral response described above.

The idea of a disturbance of membrane transport for glucose produced by the oedema finds support first of all in the experiments of Oomura *et al.* (1969). Only in the ventro-medial and lateral hypothalamus can neurones be found which change their discharge frequency in response to a change in the glucose concentration. It has not been possible to find glucose-sensitive cells either in the thalamus, the brain stem or the cerebral cortex. These findings are in agreement with our own clinical observations, that a marked hyperglycaemia always develops when there is hypothalamic involvement associated with an existing disease, process or oedema. Additional support is given to this presumed hypothetical mechanism by the preliminary results of Wesemann (1975) on brain oedema produced by cold lesions in experimental animals. It can be demonstrated by autoradiography using glucose labelled with C 14, that less glucose was available in the oedematous parts of the brain than in the control areas.

The response of the hypothalamus to the presumed intracellular hypoglycaemia or the theoretical variation of the "set point" for glucose is, as might be expected, an integrated total reaction. It consists not only in the direct encouragement of hepatic glycogenolysis, but also simultaneously in stimulation of the adrenal medulla and the pancreatic alpha-cells and the inhibition of insulin secretion. At the same time the neuro-secretion of the hypothalamic "releasing factor" as part of the integrated reaction cannot lead to a rise of HGH and ACTH or cortisol in this group of patients on account of the pre-existing damage to the pituitary gland or its stalk. Hence these hormones are not raised post-operatively in the group 7 b.

By stimulation and injury of the sympathetic neurones in the caudal brain-stem (piqure) or still more peripherally, on the other hand, effects on individual mechanisms among those mentioned are conceivable according to which part of the sympathetic pathways has been affected. This would explain the occasionally conflicting results of earlier experiments whereas the more recent experimental research on the hypothalamus supports the concepts which we have outlined.

High mean blood sugar levels were found also in patients with the full clinical neurological picture of midbrain decerebration. In this group the glucose utilization was not lowered at all as compared with the control group of post-operative patients. The highest mean concentrations of glucagon were recorded in these patients after midbrain herniation had been present for 24 hours. The mean concentration of insulin was definitely lower than in those cases with direct hypothalamic involvement and these patients also showed no adequate rise of insulin on glucose stimulation, whereas the HGH was moderately and cortisol very definitely raised. In these transverse brain-stem lesions an extreme rise of the ergotropic autonomic parameters, in the sense of a disinhibition, is characteristic. There is tachycardia, tachypnoea, hyperthermia and increased tone in the extremities. These manifestations are partly the result of a maximal increase of sympathetic tone, which is functionally cut off from the diencephalon. It was in just these groups that the highest catecholamine figures were recorded. The increased sympathetic tone leads to the disturbance of glucose metabolism already described, to an excessive rise in glucagon secretion and to inhibition of the glucose-induced insulin secretion. Without this neural control the hyperglycaemia would lead to inhibition of glucagon secretion and encouragement of insulin secretion. Its inhibition of the basal secretion determined by neural influences was evidently overriden by the extreme concentrations of glucagon in this group of patients. In several particular examples it can be shown that the rise of glucagon secretion is already present a few hours after the onset of the midbrain lesion; however, the extreme values described are only reached 24 hours after the onset of the mid-brain herniation and then persist for days and weeks along with the existing mid-brain syndrome. In most of the patients with a midbrain syndrome a paradoxical rise of HGH and cortisol was observed. It started at the moment when, after the intravenous glucose load and partition, the glucose level which was in the hyperglycaemia range began to drop. This prompt neurosecretory response resulted, as if the intracellular sugar level in the hypothalamic neurones were falling into the glucopaenic range. On account of the anatomical destruction of the neurosecretory pathways, this reaction was not observed in a group of para-hypothalamic tumours (Wiegelmann 1973).

On the other hand the incomplete medullary syndrome shows striking differences in various parameters in comparison with the mid-brain syndrome. The mean blood sugar concentration is certainly still raised, but is, however, definitely lower than in the midbrain syndrome and statistically significantly lower in comparison with the para-hypothalamic tumours. Cortisol and HGH values are raised to a similar extent as in the midbrain syndrome. On the other hand mean insulin and glucagon concentrations are significantly lower compared with those in the midbrain syndrome. Not only the basal, but also the glucose-induced insulin secretion is very small or else completely absent. The mean concentrations in these groups are lower than in all the others—even the diabetics show a still higher concentration of insulin. The glucagon concentrations are also significantly reduced and lie in the normal range or slightly above. In these groups it is evident that, in correlation with the clinical neurological findings the sympathetic tone has been reduced. The inhibition of insulin secretion is still apparent, and it appears also to involve the basal level. However glucagon secretion is no longer stimulated and therefore the neural inhibition of the basal insulin secretion can no longer be overcome. In this connexion it is difficult to decide to what extent any damage to the vagus nucleus and hence a deficiency in its stimulating influence on the insulin secretion, depending on the site or level of the lesion plays a part. The investigations of two patients with traumatic complete transverse lesions of the cervical cord did not allow us to give a clear answer to these questions. On the basis of the extent of the dislocation of the cervical spine, the neurological findings and the not modulated bradycardia one is able to assume a far-reaching disruption of sympathetic efferents with the vagus nerves intact. Raised basal insulin levels were found, as might be expected according to Porte, but however the response to glucose was only slight.

Having regard to the high glucagon and insulin values in hypothalamic lesions and the excessively high glucagon values in midbrain syndromes and considering the steep and frequently observed paradoxical HGH rise with glucose in midbrain syndromes, it would appear that somatostatin is not an essential factor in the causation of hyperglycaemia in acute lesions of the central nervous system, because administration of even very high unphysiological amounts of somatostatin in midbrain syndrome only temporarily suppresses excessive stimulation mediated via sympathetic discharge. If the latter is diminished, inhibition of both hormones by somatostatin is very marked and sustained throughout the administration. Glucose level, however, is not influenced, because both hormones are suppressed simultaneously and glycogenolysis, inhibition of insulin and increase of adrenalin secretion, all stimulated by sympathetic discharge, are not influenced by somatostatin. In addition low HGH values in these cases suggest that somatostatin is not lacking.

In patients with dissociated brain death the results are different. Hypothermia to 30 °C leads to effects on the secretion and breakdown of hormones which cannot be assessed. In investigations soon after the onset of brain death there was repeatedly, as might be expected an increase in the basal insulin level. It was a striking fact that even hours after the onset of brain death raised levels of growth hormone and of cortisol were repeatedly seen and these could be lowered to some extent by the administration of glucose. A rise of HGH secretion with arginine was sometimes observed. This is bound up with the function of the hypothalamo-pituitary system. Even when considering the existing fall in catabolism, raised concentrations of HGH and cortisol are only conceivable if one assumes partial structural and functional preservation of the hypothalamus and pituitary. It must be concluded from these findings that the group of patients with signs of brain death who are uniform from the clinical neurological and electroencephalographic standpoint show striking differences of neuroendocrinological function. In the patients described the partial preservation of hypothalamic and pituitary function is thus demonstrated, even if the course of the illness and the other findings suggest that there is a completely irreversible loss of cerebral function. With one exception all these patients have shown only a slightly raised or normal blood sugar, hours after the onset of brain death, and particularly then, if previously there was a marked hyperglycaemia associated with a hypothalamic lesion or midbrain syndrome. The abolition of the cerebral control thus resulted in a fall of the blood sugar level down to the normal range, although hypoglycaemia was not observed.

The result of the investigation of the molar insulin-glucagon quotient appeared to be of particular practical significance. While healthy subjects after a meal show a quotient of 10 to 36, it is lower in intracranial space-occupying lesions. If course is uncomplicated it rises on the first post-operative day and has returned to the pre-operative range by the seventh post-operative day. Patients with the clinical and neurological syndrome of midbrain decerebration show an extremely low quotient of 0.2 to 2. This explains the extreme wasting frequently seen in neurosurgical patients in spite of optimal high caloric feeding. The dysregulation of both hormones, which may be more clearly shown by examination of portal blood, in combination with raised cortisol values, lead to breakdown of protein and glycogen, to a sustained rise of gluconeogenesis and, because of the high excretion of catecholamines, to increased lipolysis. In spite of a high exogenous supply of calories the endogenous bodily reserves are broken up without regard to actual need, and are supplied to the organism as glucose, amino-acids (Bauer 1973) and fatty acids, although the body's requirements are already covered by the exogenous supply. Furthermore on account of the relative deficiency of insulin, the resynthesis of endogenous protein, glycogen and triglycerides is disturbed.

The pharmacokinetic approach gives some insight into the utilization of glucose in the various groups. The "transfer", *i.e.* the amount of glucose transferred in gramms per kilo body weight and per hour, with its blood level at a constant level, is reduced in all pre-operative groups as compared with the healthy. On the first post-operative day there is a rise in comsumption which has fallen again by the seventh day. It is striking on the one hand to see the very low transfer rate for glucose in pituitary tumours and anterior pituitary insufficiency, and on the other hand the high transfer rate for glucose in patients with extensor rigidity or increased extensor tonus of the extremities when associated with a midbrain syndrome (tentorial herniation).

6. Summary

The study of the literature and our own results have led to the concept of a complex control of carbohydrate metabolism by the central nervous system. This consists in the first place in the neurosecretion of releasing hormones for ACTH, *i.e.* cortisol and other glucocorticoids, for HGH and possibly also for somatostatin. In the second place, the influence appears to be neuronal via the diencephalic nuclei and structures of the sympathetic nervous system and its neurones which are frequently relayed in the brain stem and whose course is detectable even as far as the cervical cord. From there, through the peripheral portions of the sympathetic nervous system, the direct stimulation of glycogenolysis in the liver cells results as well as the promotion of glucagon secretion, the inhibition of insulin secretion in the pancreas and the stimulation of adrenaline and noradrenaline secretion in the adrenal medulla.

While the diencephalic centres of the sympathetic nervous system are in the ventro-medial nuclei, and actually in the area sympathica B of Ban, the parasympathetic centre is thought to be in the ventrolateral part of the hypothalamus. The course of the parasympathetic neurones to the vagus nuclei was demonstrated, the direct action of the vagus on glycogen synthesis in liver cells, and the neutralization of the sympathetic mediated glycogenolysis by simultaneous stimulation of the vagus was proven. Furthermore, the encouragement of insulin secretion through the branches of the vagus was also supported by animal experiments. In the hypothalamus neurosecretion and neural influences were integrated into a total response, which at its most obvious was seen in acute hypoglycaemia.

Similar to the temperature and the osmolarity, the blood sugar concentration is measured in the hypothalamus. Neurones were demonstrated in the medial and lateral hypothalamus which responded to a rise and fall of the glucose concentration with a change in the discharge rate which was dependent on the level of glucose, whereas no glucose sensitive cells could be found in any other region of the brain. In addition to the intrinsic self-regulation of the pancreas, changes in glucose concentration acting on the hypothalamus set in motion humoral and neural mechanisms which intervene in the regulation of glucose homeostasis in different ways and with varying kinetics.

To go into detail, the following results and conclusions may be drawn:

1. Even extensive chronic lesions, and displacements of the hypothalamus and other parts of the brain by intracranial space-occupying lesions, do not cause a hyperglycaemia. On the contrary there is always a slight drop in the fasting blood sugar and an increase in the sensitivity to insulin, if tumours destroy the hypothalamo-pituitary axis and lead to a deficit of HGH, ACTH and glucocorticoids or to basal values of these hormones which cannot be regulated or stimulated.

2. The highest mean hourly glucose concentrations were found after operations which lead to irritation and damage to the hypothalamus, such as the removal of craniopharyngioma, olfactory groove meningioma, tuberculum sellae meningioma and extensive suprasellar pituitary adenomas. The extent of this hyperglycaemia differed significantly from all the other post-operative groups. It could be shown from several individual observations that first of all after extensive hypothalamic lesions hypothermia and a diabetes insipidus develop, and a little later there appears an uncontrollable insulin-refractory hyperglycaemia which can be regarded as a grave prognostic sign. The hyperglycaemia associated with irritation and lesions of the hypothalamus is accompanied by a very marked hyperglucagonaemia and hyperinsulinaemia, whereas HGH and cortisol, on account of commonly existing lesions of the hypothalamo-pituitary axis show merely basal levels. Should the patient survive the irritation or lesion of the hypothalamus high blood levels of glucose, insulin and glucagon disappear after days and weeks.

Two different mechanisms are discussed as the possible cause of this striking dysregulation: the "neuronal input" of the hypothalamic cells is changed at short notice, and thus the "set point" of the glucose-sensitive neurones is also changed. The other hypothesis follows from this, that the hypothalamic neurones react in this way as though there were an intracellular glucopaenia. The cerebral oedema that may be expected after operations in the neighbourhood of the hypothalamus can lead to a disturbance of diffusion of glucose through the cell membrane and hence to an actual shortage of intracellular glucose, in spite of a high level of blood sugar. This theory can most easily explain our personal findings in the light of the literature.

3. It can be shown that a very close relationship exists between

the site of the cerebral lesion or its level in the brainstem and the extent and pattern of the dysregulation of glucose and its hormones. Patients with a midbrain decerebration also show a significant rise of the mean glucose concentration. There is an excessively raised level of glucagon in the blood, the basal insulin level is raised but there is little or no glucose-induced insulin secretion, on account of neurogenic inhibition. The maximally raised sympathetic tonus which has its result also in the excessive elevation of the other clinical para-meters, must be regarded as the pathological mechanism responsible for the hyperglycaemia, the raised glucagon secretion and the in-hibition of the reactive insulin secretion.

4. In the incomplete medullary syndrome the situation is com-pletely different. Not only the basal, but also the reactive insulin secretion is very slight or completely absent, the mean insulin levels are lower than in any other groups and even diabetics show higher mean concentrations of insulin. The glucagon levels are in the range or slightly above; the mean blood sugar concentrations are less clearly raised.

The lowest glucagon values were recorded in the healthy controls, in patients with dissociated brain death and those with high cervical complete cord lesions and hence interrupted sympathetic efferents.

5. Patients with the clinical, neurological and EEG signs of brain death showed normal to slightly raised glucose values, as a result of the failure of the central nervous influences on the blood sugar level. A few hours after the failure of cerebral function in hypothalamic lesions or the brain stem syndrome, there is consistently a fall in blood sugar from the hyperglycaemia range to the upper range of normal. On the other hand hypoglycaemia was never seen.

Raised HGH and cortisol levels in a proportion of these patients and their changes in response to glucose and arginine lead to the observation that the group of "brain dead" is not uniform, *i.e.* for some of these patients one must assume at least a partial preservation of function in the hypothalamus and pituitary, even if the clinical neurological and EEG findings, as in the rest of this group, suggest there is a failure of all brain function.

6. Pharmacokinetic studies confirm that post-operatively there is not a drop in glucose assimilation, but that actually a slight rise of utilization occurs. Thus it is not a peripheral disturbance of utiliza-tion but an increased production of glucose which accounts for the mild hyperglycaemia which is seen after operations on intracranial space-occupying lesions.

Investigations regarding the transfer, *i.e.* the turnover of glucose per kg body weight and per hour, show the lowest value in patients with pituitary tumours and anterior pituitary insufficiency. The highest values are recorded in patients with increased extensor tonus and extensor spasms, associated with a midbrain syndrome and a tentorial pressure cone. A slight rise of turnover on the first post-operative day tends to fall by the seventh but is still detectable.

7. The molar insulin-glucagon quotient determines essentially if energy is made available in the form of glucose, free fatty acids and amino acids, or if it is stored as glycogen and fat and preserved as protein. A slight elevation of this quotient appears post-operatively in intracranial space-occupying lesions. However the quotient is extremely depressed in patients with a midbrain syndrome. Catabolism of these patients in spite of high caloric feeding, is explained by the disturbed relationship of insulin and glucagon.

8. The slight post-operative hyperglycaemia and increased insulin levels described in general surgical cases are also seen after brain operations. Even on the seventh post-operative day it is still apparent but to a slightly lesser degree.

The aim of any future investigations will be to establish if the hyperglycaemia seen in lesions at various levels of the brain is necessary to the survival of oedematous neurones, or if in view of the insulin resistance which has been demonstrated it could lead to other forms of treatment, e.g. with somatostatin or a more glucagon specific analogue. Any measures which might control the central dysregulation of the insulin glucagon quotient in the treatment of wasting catabolism in neurosurgical patients appears to be promising.

References

Abramon, M., Corvillain, J., Effect of growth hormone on tubular reabsorption of glucose and phosphate. Nature *213* (1967), 85.

Adamson, U., Cerasi, E., Wahren, J., Diabetogenic and insulin-like actions of growth hormone in man. Diabetologia *11* (1975), 329.

Alberti, K. G. M. M., Christensen, E., Iversen, J., Seyer-Hansen, K., Christensen, N. J., Hansen, A. P., Ørskov, H., Inhibition of insulin secretion by Somatostatin. Lancet Dec. *8* (1973), 1299.

Allison, S. P., Prowse, K., Chamberlain, M. J., Failure of insulin response to glucose load during operation and after myocardial infarction. Lancet *1* (1967), 478.

— Hinton, P., Chamberlain, M. J., Intravenous glucose-tolerance, insulin, and free-fatty-acid levels in burned patients. Lancet 2 (1968), 1113.

— Tomlin, P. J., Chamberlain, M. J., Some effects of anesthesia and surgery on carbohydrate and fat metabolism. Brit. J. Anaesthesiol. *41* (1969), 588.

Anand, B. K., Dua, S., Blood sugar changes induced by electrical stimulation of the hypothalamus in cat. Indian J. Med. Res. *43, 1* (1955), 123.

Anderson, E., Rioch, D. McK., Haymaker, W., Disturbances in blood sugar regulation in animals subjected to transsection on the brain stem. Acta neuroveg. *5* (1952), 132.

— Curonini, C., Critchley, M., Gellhorn, E., Lopez Prieto, R., Lunedei, A., de Morsier, G., Sturm, A., Der neurovegetative Einfluß auf den Zuckerstoffwechsel. Acta neuroveg. *9.* Wien: Springer. 1954.

Bajaj, J. S., Chhina, G. S., Mohankumar, V., Garg, S. K., Baldev Singh, Evidence for the existence of an entero-hypothalamo-insular axis. Diabetologia *11* (1975), 331.

Ban, T., The septo-preoptico-hypothalamic system and its autonomic function. Progr. Brain Res. Vol. *21 A*, pp. 1—43. Amsterdam: Elsevier. 1966.

Bargmann, W., Über die neurosekretorische Verknüpfung von Hypothalamus und Neurohypophyse. Z. Zellforschung *34* (1949), 610.

— Neurosekretion. Int. Rev. Cytol. *19* (1966), 183.

— Das neurosekretorische Zwischenhirn-Hypophysensystem und seine synaptischen Verknüpfungen. J. Neuro-Visc. Relat. Suppl. *IX* (1969), 64.

Barris, R. W., Ingram, W. R., The effect of experimental hypothalamic lesions upon blood sugar. Am. J. Physiol. *114* (1935), 555.

Bauer, B. L., Untersuchungen zur renalen Ausscheidung von N-Metaboliten und Serumaminosäuren bei zentralen Regulationsstörungen. Hab. Schrift Giessen. 1973.

Bauer, H. G., Endocrine and metabolic conditions related to pathology in the hypothalamus: a review. J. Nerv. ment. Disease *128* (1959), 323.

Baum, D., Porte, D., jr., Adrenergic regulation of the inhibition of insulin release in hypothermia. Diabetes Suppl. I, Vol. *17* (1968), 298.

Beaser, S. B., Clinical states with decreased glucose tolerance. J. Am. Med. Ass. *199* (1967), 990.

Beattie, J., Insulin resistance following hypothalamic lesions and removal of the adrenal medulla. Brit. Med. J. *1* (1954), 1287.

— Brow, G. R., Long, C. N. H., Physiological and anatomical evidence of the existence of nerve tracts connecting the hypothalamus with spinal sympathetic centres. Proc. Royal Soc. *106* (1930), 253.

Berger, M., Berchtold, P., Wiegelmann, W., Drost, H., Zimmermann, H., Suppressibility of serum insulin in patients with insulinoma by Somatostatin (S.S.), Diazoxide, and Diphenylhydantoin (DPH). Diabetologia *11* (1975), 332.

Bernard, C., Chiens rendus diabétiques. Compt. Rend. Soc. Biol. *1* (1849), 60.

Bernt, E., Lachenicht, R., Methoden der Enzymatischen Analyse. Bd. *II*, 1260. Hans Ulrich Bergmeyer. 1974.

Bertram, Otto, Hormonale (zerebral-hypophysäre) Blutzuckerregulation. In: Die Zuckerkrankheit. Stuttgart: G. Thieme. 1963.

Boehm, R., Hoffmann, F. A., Beiträge zur Kenntnis des KH-Stoffwechsels. 4. Abhandl. Arch. Exp. Pathol. Pharmak. *8* (1878), 422.

Böttger, I., Schlein, E. M., Faloona, G. R., Knochel, J. P., Unger, R. H., The effect of exercise on glucagon secretion. J. Clin. Endocr. Metab. *35*, Nr. 1 (1972), 117.

Booth, D. A., Doons, E. E., Miller, N. E., Blood glucose responses to electrical stimulation of the hypothalamic feeding area. Physiol. Behavior *4* (1969), 991.

Britton, S. W., Studies on the conditions of activity in endocrine glands. XVII. The nervous control of insulin secretion. Am. J. Physiol. *74* (1925), 291.

Brücke, F., Kaindl, F., Mayer, H., Über die Veränderung in der Zusammensetzung des Nebennierenmarkinkretes bei elektrischer Reizung des Hypothalamus. Arch. Int. Pharmacodyn. *88*, Nr. 4 (1952), 407.

Byrow, F. B., Russell, D. S., Ependymal cyst of the third ventricle associated with diabetes mellitus. Lancet *2* (1932), 278.

Campfield, L. A., personal report 1975.

— Girardier, L., Nerve terminal norepinephrine uptake in collagenase isolated perfused rat islets. Diabetologia *11* (1975), 335.

— Renold, A. E., The effects of physiological concentrations of norepinephrine and epinephrine on insulin secretion. Diabetologia *11* (1975), 335.

Cannon, W. B., Hoskins, R. G., The effects of asphyxia, hyperpnoe and sensory stimulation on adrenal secretion. Am. J. Physiol. *29* (1911), 274.

— McIver, M. A., Bliss, S. W., Studies on the conditions of activity in endocrine glands. XIII. A sympathetic and adrenal mechanism. Am. J. Physiol. *69* (1924), 46.

— Newton, H. F., Bright, E. M., Menkin, V., Moore, R. M., Some aspects of the physiology of animals surviving complete exclusion of sympathetic nerve impulses. Am. J. Physiol. *89* (1929), 84.

Carraway, R., Leeman, S. E., The isolation of a new hypotensive peptide from bovine hypothalami. Fed. Proc. *30* (1971), 215.

— Demers, L., Leeman, S., Hyperglycemic effect of a hypothalamic peptide. Fed. Proc. *32* (1973), 211.

Carroll, K. F., Nestel, P. J., Diurnal variation in glucose tolerance and in insulin secretion in man. Diabetes *22* (1973), 333.

Carstens, M., Die Begutachtung des Zuckerkranken. Ärztl. Wschr. *45/46* (1949), 705.

Cerasi, E., Luft, R., Further studies on healthy subjects with low and high insulin response to glucose infusion. Acta Endocrin. *55* (1967), 305.

Chieri, R. A., Farina, J. M. S., Halperin, J., Basabe, J. C., Effect of cephalic glucose infusion on insulin secretion. Diabetologia 11 (1975), 175.

Conard, V., Mesure de l'assimilation du glucose. Acta Gastro-Enterol. Belgica XVIII (1955), 656.

Cori, C. F., Cori, G. T., The influence of epinephrine and insulin on the carbohydrate metabolism of rats in the postabsorptive state. J. Biol. Chem. LXXIX, No. 1 (1928), 321.

Creutzfeldt, W., Gastrointestinale Hormone und Insulinsekretion. Niedersächs. Ärztebl. 12 (1974), 450.

D'Amour, M. C., Keller, A. D., Blood sugar studies following hypophysectomy and experimental lesions of hypothalamus. Proc. Soc. Experim. Biol. Med. 30 (1933), 1157.

Davis, L., Cleveland, D., Ingram, W. R., Carbohydrate metabolism. Arch. Neurol. Psych. 33 (1935), 592.

Ditschuneit, H., Effect of growth hormone on metabolism. Vortrag 20. Symp. Dtsch. Ges. Endokrin. Tübingen (1974).

Donhoffer, C., McLeod, J. J. R., Studies in the nervous control of carbohydrate metabolism. I. The position of the centre. Proc. Royal Soc. 110 (1932), 125.

— — Studies in the nervous control of carbohydrate metabolism. II. The chemical changes set up in the body during decerebration hyperglycemia. Proc. Royal Soc. 110 (1932), 141.

— — Studies in the nervous control of carbohydrate metabolism. III. The nature of the mechanism of the nerve control. Proc. Royal Soc. 110 (1932), 158.

Dost, F. H., Gladtke, E., Hattingberg, M. v., Rind, H., Biokinetische Normwerte bei der intravenösen Glukosebelastung. Klin. Wschr. 46, 9 (1968), 503.

Duncombe, W. G., Klin. Chem. Acta IX (1964), 122.

Duner, H., The influence of the blood glucose level on the secretion of adrenaline and noradrenaline from the suprarenal. Acta Physiol. Scand. 28, Suppl. 102 (1953), 36.

Edwards, A. V., Silver, M., The glycogenolytic response to stimulation of the splanchnic nerves in adrenalectomized calves. J. Physiol. 211 (1970), 109.

Engelhardt, F., Die anatomischen Zwischenhirn-adenohypophysären Beziehungen. Verhandl. Dtsch. Ges. Inn. Med. 71. Kongr., 27—42. München (1965).

— Pituitary, hypothalamus and central nervous regulation. In: Modern aspects of neurosurgery (Pia, H. W., Grote, E., Mundinger, F., Gleave, J. R. W., eds.), Vol. I, pp. 3—10. Amsterdam: Excerpta Medica. 1971.

Erbslöh, F., Das ZNS bei Leberkrankheiten. In: Handbuch der speziellen Anatomie und Histologie 35/2, p, 1645. Berlin-Göttingen-Heidelberg: Springer. 1958.

— Veränderungen des ZNS bei Erkrankungen des Magen-Darm-Traktes und der Bauchspeicheldrüse. Handbuch der Pathologischen Anatomie XIII/2, 1699 (1958).

— Das ZNS bei Krankheiten der Drüsen mit innerer Sekretion. In: Handbuch der Pathologischen Anatomie XIII/2 (1958), 1740.

— Hillesheim, H. R., Der Glukoseverbrauch des Hirns und seine Abhängigkeit von der Leber. Arch. Psych. Nervenkrankh. 196 (1958), 611.

Esterhuizen, A. C., Lever, J. D., Pancreatic islet cells in the normal and $COCl_2$-treated guinea-pig. A fine structural study. J. Endocrin. 23 (1961), 243.

— Spriggs, T. L., Lever, J. D., Nature of islet-cell innervation in the cat pancreas. Diabetes 17 (1968), 33.

— Howell, S. L., Ultrastructure of the A-cells of cat islets of Langerhans following sympathetic stimulation of glucagon secretion. J. Cell. Biol. 46 (1970), 593.

Exton, J. H., Robinson, G. A., Sutherland, E. W., Park, C. R., Studies on the role of Adenosine 3'-5'-Monophosphate in the hepatic actions of glucagon and catecholamines. J. Biol. Chem. 246, 6166. Baltimore (1971 a).

Ezdinli, E. Z., Javid, R., Owens, G., Sokal, J. E., Effect of high spinal cord section on epinephrine hyperglycemia. Am. J. Physiol. 214 (1968), 1019.

Falta, W., Zentralnervensystem und Diabetes. In: Die Zuckerkrankheit, S. 211. Berlin und Wien: Urban & Schwarzenberg. 1944.

Feyrter, S., Über das Inselorgan und seine vegetative Innervation. Acta neuroveg. 9, 44. Wien: Springer. 1954.

Findlay, J. A., Gill, J. R., Lever, J. D., Randle, P. J., Spriggs, T. L. B., Increased insulin output following stimulation of the vagal supply to the perfused rabbit pancreas. J. Anat. 104 (1969), 580.

Förster, E., Holldorf, A. W., Falk, H., Probleme der Stoffwechselregulation in der Leber. II. Regulationsmechanismen im Kohlenhydratstoffwechsel. Acta hepato-splenol. 15, 257. Stuttgart 1968.

Frerichs, H., Creutzfeldt, W., Physiologische und pharmakologische Beeinflussung der Insulinsekretion. Med. Klin. 66 (1971), 1039.

Frohman, L. A., The hypothalamus and metabolic control. Pathobiol. Ann. 2—25 (1971).

— Ezdinli, E. Z., Javid, R., Effect of vagotomy and vagal stimulation on insulin secretion. Diabetes 16 (1967), 443.

— Bernardis, L. L., Growth hormone and insulin levels in weanling rats with ventromedial hypothalamic lesions. Endocr. 82 (1968), 1125.

— — Kant, K. J., Hypothalamic stimulation of growth hormone secretion. Science 162 (1968), 580.

— — Effect of hypothalamic stimulation on plasma glucose, insulin, and glucagon levels. Am. J. Physiol. 221, No. 6 (1971), 1596.

— Goldman, J. K., Bernardis, L. L., Studies of insulin sensitivity in vivo in weanling rats with hypothalamic obesity. Metabolism 21, No. 12 (1972), 1133.

Fussgänger, R. D., Laube, H., Pfeiffer, E. F., Das isoliert verfundierte Pankreas. Therap. Berichte Bayer-Leverkusen 1 (1974), 77.

Ganon, W. S., Neuroendokrine Mechanismen. In: Neuroendocrinology, Vol. 1, p. 1. New York-London: Academic Press. 1966.

Garcia, S. D., Rosselin, G., Effect of Somatostatin on insulin biosynthesis. Diabetologia 11 (1975), 339.

Gellhorn, E., Cortell, R., Feldman, J., The effect of emotion, sham rage, and hypothalamic stimulation on the vago-insulin system. Am. J. Physiol. 133 (1941), 532.

Gentes, M., Note sur les terminaisons nerveuses des ilots de Langerhans du pancréas. Compt. Rend. Soc. Biol. 54 (1902), 202.

Geser, C. A., Die Verwertung von Kohlenhydraten in Streß-Situationen. Die Infusionstherapie 1, Nr. 3 (1974), 215.

— Schultis, K., Diedrichson, W., Das Seruminsulin in der postoperativen Phase unter parenteraler Ernährung. Med. und Ernährg. 11 (1970), 82.

Gissel, H., Stoffwechselstörungen nach Hirntraumen. Zbl. Chir. J. 60, Nr. 1—17 (1933), 765.

Gladtke, E., Hattingberg, H. M. v., Pharmakokinetik. Berlin-Heidelberg-New York: Springer. 1973.

Gottstein, U., Held, K., Insulinwirkung auf den menschlichen Hirnmetabolismus von Stoffwechselgesunden und Diabetikern. Klin. Wschr. 45 (1967), 18.

Grabner, W., Daniel, U., Fischer, K., Phillip, J., Zuverlässigere Diabetes-Therapie durch Sekretionstyp-Analyse. Med. Tribune 44 (1974), 15.

Grafe, E., Über die nervöse Regulation des organischen Stoffwechsels und ihre Störungen. Verhandl. Ges. Dtsch. Nervenärzte, 22. Jahresversammlung, S. 6—27. Berlin: F. C. W. Vogel. 1935.

Green, J. D., Neural pathways to the hypophysis: anatomical and functional. In: The hypothalamus. Springfield, Ill.: Ch. C Thomas. 1969.

Guder, W. G., Schmidt, U., Intrarenal localization of gluconeogenesis. Diabetologia 11 (1975), 345.

Hagen, E., Zentralnervöse Regulationssysteme. In: Physiologie und Pathophysiologie des vegetativen Nervensystems (Monnier, M., Hrsg.), Bd. I, S. 16—51. Stuttgart: Hippokrates Verlag. 1963.

Hallpike, J. F., Claveria, L. E., Cohen, N. M., Lascelles, P. T., Glucose tolerance and plasma insulin levels in subarachnoid hemorrhage. Brain 94/1 (1971), 151.

Halmagyi, D. F. G., Neering, I. R., Lazarus, L., Young, J. D., Pullin, J., Plasmaglucagon in experimental post hemorrhagic shock. J. Trauma 9 (1969), 320.

Harris, G. W., George, R., Neurohumoral control of the adenohypophysis and the regulation of the secretion of TSH, ACTH, and growth hormone. In: The hypothalamus. Springfield, Ill.: Ch. C Thomas. 1969.

Hasselblatt, A., Stoffwechselwirkungen der Katecholamine. In: Handbuch der Inneren Medizin (Oberdisse, K., Hrsg.), Teil II A: Stoffwechselkrankheiten, 5. Aufl., Bd. 7, S. 503. Berlin-Heidelberg-New York: Springer. 1975.

Hattingberg, H. M. v., Mathematische Verfahren zur Auswertung von pharmakokinetischen Untersuchungen. Arzneimittel-Forschung (Drug Res.) 23, Nr. 11 a (1973), 1646.

— Cornelius, U., Gladtke, E., Der Glukoseumsatz bei Kindern mit Acetonurie. Klin. Wschr. 7, Nr. 17 (1969), 909.

— Gladtke, E., Dost, F. H., Die Differenzierung der pathologischen Kohlenhydrattoleranz. Dtsch. med. Wschr. 95, Nr. 7 (1970), 349.

— Dost, F. H., Gladtke, E., Besonderheiten der Biokinetik der Glukose bei normalen und übergewichtigen Neugeborenen. Klin. Wschr. 51 (1973), 455.

Hautecouverture, M., Basdevant, A., Slama, G., Tchobroutsky, G., Diurnal variations in plasma glucose and insulin levels after i.v. Glucagon and Arginine infusion in men and women. Diabetologia 11 (1975), 347.

Heldt, H. W., Morphologische und funktionelle Kompartimentierung des Zellstoffwechsels. In: Physiologie des Menschen (Gauer, Kramer, Jung, Hrsg.), Bd. 1, S. 225—269. München-Berlin-Wien: Urban & Schwarzenberg. 1972.

Hess, W. R., Die funktionelle Organisation des vegetativen Nervensystems. Basel: B. Schwabe. 1948.

Himms-Hagen, J., Sympathetic regulation of metabolism. Pharmak. Rev. 19, Nr. 3 (1967), 367.

— Effect of catecholamines on metabolism. In: Catecholamines (Blaschko, H., Muscholl, E., eds.). Berlin-Heidelberg-New York: Springer. 1972.

Himsworth, R. L., Hypothalamic control of adrenaline secretion in response to insufficient glucose. J. Physiol. 206 (1970), 411.

Hinton, P., Allison, S. P., Littlejohn, S., Lloyd, J., Insulin and glucose to reduce catabolic response to injury in burned patients. Lancet 17 (1971), 767.

Högler, F., Die zentral-nervöse Blutzuckerregulation. In: Diabetes mellitus, S. 115 —141. München-Berlin-Wien: Urban & Schwarzenberg. 1950.

Hoff, F., Die hypothalamische Steuerung des Hypophysenvorderlappens. Verhandl. Dtsch. Ges. Inn. Med., 71. Kongr., S. 15—27. München 1965.

Hoff, H., Der Hypothalamus, seine Anatomie, Physiologie und Pathologie. Acta neuroveg. 1, 123. Wien: Springer. 1950.

Holldorf, A. W., personal report 1974.

— Förster, E., Falk, H., Probleme der Stoffwechselregulation in der Leber. I. Allgemeine Grundlagen der Regulation von Stoffwechselvorgängen. Acta Hepato-Splenol. *15*, Nr. 3 (1968), 129.

— — — Probleme der Stoffwechselregulation in der Leber. IV. Über den Wirkungsmechanismus einiger Hormone. Acta Hepato-Splenol. *15*, Nr. 6 (1968), 361.

Horecker, B. L., Stoffwechselwege der Kohlenhydrate: Ihre Regulierung und psychische Bedeutung. Vortrag an der Med. Abtlg. der Kyoto-Univ. Japan vom 29. September 1967.

Houssay, B. A., Biasotti, A., Pankreasdiabetes und Hypophyse beim Hund. Pflügers Arch. Ges. Physiol. *227* (1931), 664.

— — Rietti, C. T., Action diabétogène de l'extrait ante-hypophysaire. Compt. rend. hebdomadaires de la Société de biologie. Ann. 1932, Tome III, 479. Paris: Masson et Cie. 1932.

Howard, J. M., Studies of the absorption and metabolism of glucose following injury. Ann. Surgery *141*, No. 3 (1955), 321.

Hustvedt, B. D., Haug, A., Løvø, A., Hepatic triglyceride secretion and free fatty acid flux in vivo after ventromedial hypothalamic lesions. Diabetologia *11* (1975), 351.

Idahl, L. A., Effect of anoxia on the glycolytic flux in pancreatic beta-cells. Diabetologia *11* (1975), 351.

— Martin, J. M., Stimulation of insulin release by a ventro-lateral hypothalamic factor. J. Endocr. *51* (1971), 601.

Iversen, J., Adrenergic receptors and the secretion of glucagon and insulin from the isolated perfused canine pancreas. Clin. Invest. *52* (1973), 2102.

— Further characterization of the inhibitory effect of somatostatin on insulin and glucagon release from the isolated perfused canine pancreas. Diabetologia *11* (1975), 352.

Johnston, J. D. A., The metabolic and endocrine response to injury: a review. Brit. J. Anaesthesiol. *45* (1973), 252.

Joost, H. G., Lenzen, S., Beckmann, J., Hasselblatt, A., Inhibition of insulin and glucagon release by cyproheptadine in the rat. Diabetologia *11* (1975), 353.

Jungmann, E., Bach, G., Böhmer, D., Eckardt, D., Haas, I., The effects of exercise, catecholamines and the blockade of adrenergic beta-receptors on the assimilation of glucose. Diabetologia *11* (1975), 353.

Kaneto, A., Miki, E., Kosaka, K., Okinaka, S., Nakao, K., Effects of stimulation of the cingulate gyrus on insulin secretion. Endocrinology *77* (1965), 617.

— Kosaka, K., Nakao, K., Effects of stimulation of the vagus nerve on insulin secretion. Endocrinology *80*, Jan.-June (1967).

— Kajinuma, H., Kosaka, K., Nakao, K., Stimulation of insulin secretion by parasympathomimetic agents. Endocrinology *83* (1968), 651.

Karakash, C., Hustvedt, B., LeMarchand, Y., Jean-Renaud, B., Hyperinsulinemia following ventro-medial hypothalamus lesions: possible consequences upon liver metabolism. Diabetologia *11* (1975), 354.

Kern, H. F., Hofmann, H. V., Kern, D., Licht- und elektronenmikroskopische Untersuchung der Langerhans'schen Inseln von Nutria (Myocaster coypus), mit besonderer Berücksichtigung der neuroinsulären Komplexe. Z. Zellforschung *113* (1971), 216.

— Grube, D., Comparative structure and innervation of pancreatic islets. Endocrinology Proc. IV. Internat. Congr. of Endocr. Washington, 18–24 June 1972. Amsterdam: Excerpta Medica. 1972.

Keymolen-Jardini, V., Mouawad, E., Claeys-DeClerq, P., Laere, E. van, Levin, S., Borkowski, A., Glucose metabolism in traumatic brain injury. Acta Endocr. Nov., 1 (1973).

Killeffer, F. A., Stern, W. E., Chronic effects of hypothalamic injury. Arch. Neurol. 22 (1970), 419.

King, L. R., Knowles, H. C., jr., McLaurin, R. L., Lewis, H. P., Glucose tolerance and plasma insulin in cranial trauma. Ann. Surgery 173 (1971), 337.

Knick, B., Umdenken über Kohlenhydrate. Ärztl. Praxis XXVI, Nr. 31 (1974), 1527.

Kobayashi, K., Electron microscope studies of the Langerhans islets in the toad pancreas. Arch. Histol. Japon. 26 (1966), 439.

— Fujita, T., Fine structure of mammalian and avian pancreatic islets with special reference to D-cells and nervous elements. Z. Zellforschung 100 (1969), 340.

Koch, G., Vergleichende Untersuchungen über das Blutglukose- und Plasmainsulin-verhalten an traumatisierten Kaninchen. Bruns Beitr. Klin. Chirurgie 221 (1974), 158.

Kracht, J., Wirkungen von Wachstumshormon auf die Langerhans'schen Inseln des Rattenpankreas. Naturwissenschaften 40 (1953), 607.

Kreyszig, E., Statistische Methoden und ihre Anwendungen. Göttingen: Vandenhoeck u. Ruprecht. 1968.

Krieger, D. T., Allen, W., Rizo, F., Krieger, H. P., Plasma corticosteroid levels. J. Clin. Endocr. Metabol. 32 (1971), 226.

Krulich, L., Hypothalamic regulation of the secretion of the growth hormone. Acta Endocr. Suppl. 184 (1974), 179.

Kühl, C., Andersen, O., Lindkaer Jensen, S., Vagn Nielsen, O., The effect of ethanol on serum insulin concentration in portal hepatic and peripheral venous blood. Diabetologia 11 (1975), 357.

Kurotsu, T., Kuritani, T., Ban, T., Studies on the changes of pancreatic islets induced by the electrical stimulation of the hypothalamus of normal and adrenalectomized rabbits. Med. J. Osaka Univ. 8 (1957), 111.

Lammers, H. J., The neuronal connexions of the hypothalamic neurosecretory nuclei in mammals. J. Neuro-Visc. Rel. Suppl. IX (1969), 311.

Landgraf, R., Weißmann, A., Hörl, R., Landgraf-Leurs, M. M. C., Is prolactin a diabetogenic hormone? Diabetologia 11 (1975), 352.

Lange, R., Zur Kenntnis der Feinstruktur der Langerhans'schen Inseln von hungernden Fröschen. Z. Zellforschung 65 (1965), 176.

Lausberg, G., Zentrale Störungen der Temperaturregulation. Acta neurochir. (Wien) Suppl. XIX (1972).

Lefebvre, P., Luyckx, A., Glucagon and catecholamines. In: Glucagon (Lefebvre, P., Unger, R., eds.), pp. 175—180. Oxford-New York- Toronto-Sydney-Braunschweig: Pergamon-Press. 1972.

Legg, P. G., The fine structure and innervation of the beta and delta cells in the islet of Langerhans of the cat. Z. Zellforschung 80 (1967), 307.

Leipert, T., Stoffwechsel und vegetative Regulation. Acta neuroveg. 1, 52—73. Wien: Springer. 1950.

Lenzen, S., Joost, H. G., Beckmann, J., Hasselblatt, A., Selective and reversible inhibition of glucose-induced insulin secretion caused by thyroxine treatment. Diabetologia 11 (1975), 359.

Leuthardt, F., Der Kohlenhydratstoffwechsel. Lehrbuch der Physiologischen Chemie, S. 279—354. Berlin: Walter de Gruyter & Co. 1963.

Levine, R., Wirkungsmechanismen des Insulins: Derzeitiger Stand der Forschung. Verhandl. Dtsch. Ges. Inn. Med., 76. Kongr. München, S. 1—13. München: J. F. Bergmann. 1970.

Lindsey, A., Santeusanio, F., Braaten, J., Faloona, G. R., Unger, R. H., Pancreatic alphacell function in trauma. J. Am. Assoc. 227 (1974), 757.

Lindsey, C. A., Faloona, G. R., Unger, R. H., Plasma glucagon in nonketotic hyperosmolar coma. J. Am. Med. Assoc. 229 (1974), 1771.

Lorenz, R., Kriterien der Hirntätigkeit in lebensbedrohten Zuständen — ein Beitrag zur Frage des zentralen Todes. Acta neurochir. (Wien) Suppl. XX (1969), 309.

— Wirkungen intrakranieller raumfordernder Prozesse auf den Verlauf von Blutdruck und Pulsfrequenz. Acta neurochir. (Wien) Suppl. XX (1973).

Loubatières, A., Pharmacological aspects of insulin secretion. Diabetes Proc. 7th Congr. Internat. Diabetes Federat. 137—158 (1971).

Lübken, W., Neurovegetative Regulation. Aus: Diabetes mellitus, S. 25—26. Stuttgart: Hippokrates-Verlag. 1960.

Luft, R., Cerasi, E., Human growth hormone as a regulator of blood glucose concentration and as a diabetogenic substance. Acta Endocr. Suppl. CXXIV (1967), 9.

Luyckx, A. S., Sécrétion de l'insuline et de glucagon. Etude clinique et expérimentale. Contribution du système nerveux autonome ortho-sympathique à l'élévation de la glucagonémie au course de la mage forcée chez le vent. Paris: Masson & Cie. 1974.

— Lefebvre, P. J., Influence of Somatostatin (SRIF) on nicotinic acid-induced changes in blood glucose (BG), free fatty acid (FFA), glucagon (PG) growth hormone (GH) and Cortisol (Co) in diabetic subjects. Diabetologia 11 (1975), 360.

Maccario, M., Neurological dysfunction associated with nonketotic hyperglycemia. Arch. Neurol. 19 (1968), 525.

Malaisse, W. J., Insulin secretion: multifactorial regulation for a single process of release. Diabetologia 9 (1973), 167.

— Sener, A., Levy, J., Fasting-induced pression of key glycolytic enzymes in pancreatic islets. Diabetologia 11 (1975), 361.

Malherbe, C., et al., Phenytoin (Diphenylhydantoin) und Insulinsekretion. Arzneimittelbrief, unabhängiges Informationsblatt für den Arzt 6, Nr. 5 (1972), 32.

Marguth, F., Differentialdiagnostik der Geschwülste im Bereich des Türkensattels. Dtsch. med. Wschr. 89, Nr. 39 (1964), 1839.

Marliss, E. B., Girardier, L., Seydoux, J., Wollheim, C. B., Kanazawa, Y., Orci, L., Renold, A. E., Porte, D., jr., Glucagon release induced by pancreatic nerve stimulation in the dog. J. Clin. Invest. 52 (1973) 1246.

Marschner, I., Dobry, H., Erhardt, F., Landersdorfer, T., Popp, B., Ringel, C., Scriba, P. C., Berechnung radioimmunologischer Meßwerte mittels Spline-Funktionen. Ärztl. Lab. 6 (1974), 184.

— Erhardt, F., Scriba, P. C., Calculation of the radioimmunoassay standard curve by "spline function". Internat. Atomic Energy Agency 1 (1974), 111, Wien.

Martin, J. M., Mok, C. C., Penfold, J., Howard, N. J., Crowne, D., Hypothalamic stimulation of insulin release. J. Endocr. 58 (1973), 681.

Matzkies, F., Berg, G., Heid, H., Improved metabolic clearance of glucose during infusion of a carbohydrate mixture containing glucose, xylit, and fructose. Diabetologia 11 (1975), 362.

McNamara, J. J., Molot, M., Stremple, J. F., Sleemann, H. K., Hyperglycemia response to trauma in combat casualties. J. Trauma 11/4 (1971), 337.

Mehnert, H., Förster, H., Stoffwechselkrankheiten. Stuttgart: G. Thieme. 1970.
— Schöffling, K. (Hrsg.), Diabetologie in Klinik und Praxis. Stuttgart: G. Thieme. 1974.
Mellanby, J., The influence of the nervous system on glycemia and glycosuria. J. Physiol. *53* (1919/20), 1.
Misbin, R. J., Edgar, P. J., Lockwood, D. H., Adrenergic regulation of insulin secretion during fasting in normal subjects. Diabetes *19* (1970), 688.
Molinatti, G. M., Massara, F., Strumia, E., Pennisi, F., Scassellati, G. A., Vancheri, L., Radioimmunoassay of human growth hormone. J. Nucl. Biol. Med. *13* (1969), 26.
Morgan, L. O., Vonderrahe, A. R., Malone, E. F., Pathological changes in the hypothalamus in diabetes mellitus. J. Nerv. Ment. Disease *85*, No. 2 (1937), 125.
Morrhouse, J. A., Chochinov, R. H., Perlman, K., Alanine turnover and disposal in healthy subjects. Diabetologia *11* (1975), 364.
Mortimer, C. H., Turnbridge, W. M. G., Carr, D., Yeomans, L., Lind, T., Coy, D. H., Bloom, S. R., Kastin, A., Mallinson, C. N., Besser, G. M., Schally, A. V., Hall, R., Effects of growth-hormone release-inhibiting hormone on circulating glucagon, insulin, and growth-hormone in normal, diabetic, acromegalic, and hypopituitary patients. Lancet (1974), 697.
Mouawad, E., Laere, E. van, Troubles de la glycémie chez les traumatisés crâniens. Neuro-Chirurgie *19*, No. 5 (1973), 456.
— — Traumatisme crânien et diabète sucre attitude thérapeutique. Extrait des Annales de l'Anestésiologie française *XV*, Nr. 4 (1974), 335.
Munger, B., The histology, psychochemistry, and ultrastructure of pancreatic islet alpha-cells. In: Glucagon (Lefebvre, P., Unger, R. H., eds.). Oxford-Toronto-New York-Sydney-Braunschweig: Pergamon Press. 1972.
Murphy, B. E. P., Some studies of the protein-binding of steroids and their application to the routine micro and ultramicro measurement of various steroids in body fluids by competitive protein-binding radio-assay. J. Clin. Endocr. Metabol. *27*, No. 7 (1967), 973.
— Protein binding and the assay of nonantigenic hormones. Progr. in Hormone Res. *25* (1969), 563.
— Engelberg, W., Pattee, C. J., Simple method for the determination of plasma corticoids. J. Endocr. Metabol. *23* (1963), 293.
Nieschlag, E., Wombacher, H., Kroeger, F. J., Overzier, C., Die Bestimmung von Wachstumshormon (HGH) als Diagnostikum bei chromophoben und eosinophilen Adenomen der Hypophyse. Klin. Wschr. *49*, Nr. 20 (1971), 1138.
Nitsche, J., Praktische Mathematik. Mannheim: Bibliographisches Institut AG. 1960.
Oberdisse, K., Befunde am vegetativen System bei Schädeltraumen. Zbl. Neurochir. *10* (1950), 69.
— Kohlenhydratstoffwechsel bei organischen Erkrankungen im Sellabereich. Dtsch. Arch. klin. Med. *198* (1951), 257.
— (Hrsg.), Diabetes mellitus. In: Handbuch der Inneren Medizin. 5. Aufl. Bd. 7. Stoffwechselkrankheiten Teil II A. Berlin-Heidelberg-New York: Springer. 1975.
— Paraskevopoulous, J. N., Über die Beeinflussung der Zuckerausscheidungsschwelle durch den Hypophysenvorderlappen. Z. exper. Med. *108* (1941), 317.
— Rauser, E., Insulinbelastung bei frischen gedeckten Hirnverletzungen. Klin. Wschr. *27*, Nr. 17/18 (1949), 316.
— Tönnis, W., Pathophysiologie, Klinik und Behandlung der Hypophysenadenome. Ergebnisse der Inneren Medizin und Kinderheilkunde. 4. Band, S. 975. Berlin-Göttingen-Heidelberg: Springer. 1953.

Oomura, Y., Kimura, K., Ooyama, H., Maeno, T., Iki, M., Kuniyoshi, M., Reciprocal activities of the ventro-medial and lateral hypothalamic areas of cats. Science *143* (1964), 484.

— Ono, T., Ooyama, H., Wayner, M. J., Glucose and osmosensitive neurones of the rat hypothalamus. Nature *222* (1969), 282.

Oppenheimer, J., Abnormalities of neuroendocrine functions in man. Neuroendocrinology, Vol. II, Chapter 33, p. 665. New York-London: Academic Press. 1967.

Orsetti, A., Passebois, F., The production of insulin by isolated fragments of pancreas directly stimulated by way of their vagal fibre. Importance of the glucose concentration of the medium. Diabetologia *11* (1975), 367.

Orthner, H., Hypothalamische Krankheiten. Handbuch der speziellen pathologischen Anatomie und Histologie XII/5, S. 543. Berlin-Göttingen-Heidelberg: Springer. 1955.

— Zur Pathophysiologie hypophysär-hypothalamischer Krankheiten. Wien. med. Wschr. *108*, Nr. 5 (1958), 95.

Pausch, H., Psychisches Trauma und Diabetes mellitus. Klin. Wschr. *46*, Nr. 17 (1951), 527.

Penfield, W., The influence of the diencephalon and hypophysis upon general autonomic function. Can. Med. Assoc. J. *XXX*, No. 6 (1934), 589.

Pensa, A., Osservazioni sulla distribuzione dei vasi sanguigni e dei nervi nel pancreas. Internat. Monatsschrift f. Anat. & Physiol. Bd. XXII, S. 116. Leipzig: G. Thieme. 1905.

Pfanzagel, J., Allgemeine Methodenlehre der Statistik. Sammlung Göschen, Bd. 747, Berlin 1966.

Pfeiffer, E. F., Wachstumshormon und Insulinsekretion: Die Verhältnisse unter normalen und pathologischen Bedingungen. In: Wachstumshormon und Wachstumsstörungen. Das Cushing-Syndrom. 11. Symp. der Dtsch. Ges. f. Endokr. in Düsseldorf 1964, S. 41—55. Berlin-Göttingen-Heidelberg-New York: Springer. 1965.

— Die Insulinsekretion — Stimulierung und Hemmung. Verhdlg. Dtsch. Ges. Inn. Med. (Schlegel, B., Hrsg.), 76. Kongr. Wiesbaden 1969, S. 32—51, 1969.

— Fortschritte der Diabetologie. Sonderdruck aus: Therapiewoche *21* (1971), 553 (1—12).

— (Hrsg.), Handbuch des Diabetes mellitus. Pathophysiologie und Klinik. München: Verlag Lehmann. 1971.

— Obesity, islet function and diabetes mellitus. Acta Endocr. Suppl. *173* (1973), 181.

— Fussgänger, R., Hinz, M., Raptis, S., Schleyer, M., Straub, K., Extrapancreatic hormones and insulin secretion. Diabetes. Proc. of the 7th Congr. of the Internat. Diabetes Federation. Exc. Med. 460 (1971).

Pia, H. W., Die Schädigung des Hirnstammes bei den raumfordernden Prozessen des Gehirns. Acta neurochir. (Wien) Suppl. IV. Wien: Springer. 1957.

— Hirnstammsyndrome bei zentraler Dysregulation. Seara Med. Neurocir. *1*, No. 5 (1973), 541.

Porte, D., jr., A receptor mechanism for the inhibition of insulin release by epinephrine in man. J. Clin. Inv. *46* (1967), 86.

— Sympathetic regulation of insulin secretion. Arch. Intern. Med. *123* (1969), 252.

— Graber, A. L., Kuzuya, T., Williams, R. H., The effect of epinephrine on immunoreactive insulin levels in man. J. Clin. Inv. *45* (1966), 228.

Rabinowitz, D., Merimee, T. J., Burgess, J. A., Growth hormone—insulin interaction. Diabetes *15*, No. 12 (1966), 905.

Raisman, G., Neural connexions of the hypothalamus. Brit. Bull. 22, No. 3 (1966) 197.

Raptis, S., Dollinger, H. C., Schlegel, W., Nadjafi, A. S., Portal and peripheral blood concentrations of insulin and exocrine pancreatic secretion in response to pure (99%) cholecystokinin-pancreozymin (CCK) in man. Diabetologia 11 (1975), 371.

Reaven, G. M., Ginsberg, H., Javorski, C., Kimmerling, G., Olefsky, J., Mechanism of insulin resistance in diabetes. Diabetologia 11 (1975), 372.

Reeves, A. G., Plum, F., Hyperphagia, rage, and dementia accompanying a ventro-medial hypothalamic neoplasm. Arch. Neurol. 20 (1969), 616.

Reiss, E., Experimenteller Beitrag zur Frage der zentral-nervösen Steuerung des Kohlenhydratstoffwechsels. Acta neuroveg. 1, 40. Wien: Springer. 1950.

Robbers, H., Der renale Diabetes. Klinik der Zuckerausscheidungen bei normalem Blutzucker. Stuttgart: Wissenschaftl. Verlagsanstalt. 1946.

Robertson, R. P., Porte, D., jr., Adrenergic modulation of basal insulin secretion in man. Diabetes 22 (1973), 1.

Roch-Norland, A., Horn, R., Walaas, E., Walaas, O., Regulation of cyclic AMP dependent protein kinase in human skeletal muscle in vivo by epinephrine and insulin. Diabetologia 11 (1975), 372.

Rocha, D. M., Santeusanio, F., Faloona, G. R., Unger, R. H., Abnormal pancreatic alpha-cell function in bacterial infections. New Engl. J. Med. 288 (1973), 700.

Rosenberg, F. J., DiStefano, V., A central nervous system component of epinephrine hyperglycemia. Am. J. Physiol. 203 (1962), 782.

Ross, H., Johnston, I. D. A., Welborn, T. A., Wright, A. D., Effect of abdominal operation on glucose tolerance and serum levels of insulin, growth hormone, and hydrocortisone. Lancet 10 (1966), 563.

Rothballer, A. B., Some endocrine manifestations of central nervous system disease. Bull. New York Acad. Med. 42, No. 4 (1966), 258.

Sachs, L., Statistische Auswertungsmethoden. Berlin-Heidelberg-New York: Springer. 1969.

Samols, E., personal report 1975.

— Inhibition of glucagon secretion by diazoxide. Clin. Res. Jan. (1975).

— Marks, V., Nouvelles conceptions sur la signification fonctionnelle du glucagon. Journées Annuelles de Diabétologie de l'Hotel Drein, 43—66 (1967).

— Tyler, J. M., Kajinuma, H., Influence of the sulfonamides on pancreatic humoral secretion and evidence for an insulin-glucagon feedback system. Diabetes. Proc. 7th Congr. Internat. Diabetes Feder. Exc. Med. (1971), 636—655.

— — Marks, V., Glucagon-insulin Interrelationships. In: Glucagon (Lefebvre, P., Unger, R. H., eds.), pp. 7—25. Oxford-New York-Toronto-Sydney-Braunschweig: Pergamon Press. 1972.

Sano, K., Mayanagi, Y., Sekino, H., Ogashiva, M., Ishijima, B., Results of stimulation and destruction of the posterior hypothalamus in man. J. Neurosurg. 33 (1970), 689.

Sarcione, E. J., Sokal, J. E., Gerszi, K. E., Relation of the adrenal medulla to the hyperglycemic effect of glucagon. Endocrinology 67 (1960), 337.

Sauer, R., Szabo, I., Mathematische Hilfsmittel des Ingenieurs. Berlin-Heidelberg-New York: Springer. 1968.

Schade, J. P., A system analysis of some hypothalamic functions. In: The hypothalamus (Martini, L., Motta, M., Fraschine, F., eds.), pp. 69—82. New York: Academic Press. 1970.

Scharrer, E., Principles of neuro-endocrine integration. In: Endocrines and the central nervous system (Levine, R., ed.). Proc. of the Assoc. Dec. 6–7, 1963, pp. 1—35 (Baltimore). New York: The Williams & Wilkins Comp. 1966.

Schatz, H., A Rahman, Y., Hinz, M., Fehm, H. L., Nierle, C., Pfeiffer, E. F., Hypophysis and function of pancreatic islets. I. The influence of hypophysectomy on insulin secretion and biosynthesis of proinsulin and insulin in isolated pancreatic islets of rat. Diabetologia 9 (1973), 135.

— Katsilambros, N., Hinz, M., Voigt, K. H., Nierle, C., Pfeiffer, E. F., Hypophysis and function of pancreatic islets. II. The effect of substitution of growth hormone and corticotropin on insulin secretion and biosynthesis of proinsulin and insulin in isolated islets of hypophysectomized rats. Diabetologia 9 (1973), 140.

Schultis, K., Veränderungen im Kohlenhydrat- und Fettstoffwechsel nach Operationen und Traumata. Thesis Giessen 1971.

Scriba, P. C., Endocrinology of the hypothalamus and the pituitary gland. In: Modern aspects of neurosurgery (Kuhlendahl, H., Brock, M., LeVay, D., Weston, T. J., eds.), Vol. IV, p. 83. Amsterdam: Excerpta Medica. 1973.

— Endocrinology of the hypothalamus and the pituitary gland. In: Modern aspects of neurosurgery (Kuhlendahl, H., Brock, M., LeVay, D., Weston, T. J., eds.), Vol. IV, p. 89. Amsterdam: Excerpta Medica. 1973.

— Karg, H., Prolaktin und Endokrinologie der Mamma — Indikationen für synthetische Hypothalamushormone. Dtsch. med. Wschr. 17 (1975), 967.

Seeger, W., Atemstörungen bei intrakraniellen Massenverschiebungen. Acta neurochir. (Wien) Suppl. XVIII. Wien: Springer. 1968.

Senft, G., Hormonal control of carbohydrate and lipid metabolism and drug induced alterations. Naunyn-Schmiedebergs Archiv für Pharmakologie 259 (1967/68), 117.

— Sitt, R., Losert, W., Schultz, G., Hoffmann, M., Hemmung der Insulinsekretion durch Alpha-Rezeptoren stimulierende Substanzen. Naunyn-Schmiedebergs Archiv für Pharmakologie und exp. Pathologie 260 (1968), 309.

Shimazu, T., Glycogen synthetase activity in liver: regulation by the autonomic system. Science 156 (1967), 1256.

— Fukuda, A., Increased activities of glycogenolytic enzymes in liver after splanchnic-nerve stimulation. Science 150 (1965), 1607.

— — Ban, T., Reciprocal influence of the ventromedial and lateral hypothalamic nuclei on blood glucose level and liver glycogen content. Nature 210 (1966), 1178.

— Amakawa, A., Regulation of glycogen metabolism in liver by the autonomic nervous system. II. Neural control of glycogenolytic enzymes. Biochim. Biophys. Acta 165 (1968), 349.

Shorr, S. S., Bloom, F. E., Fine structure of islet-cell innervation in the pancreas of normal and Alloxan-treated rats. Z. Zellforschung 103 (1970), 12.

Shull, K. H., Mayer, J., Experimental hyperglycemic states not primarily due to a lack of insulin. Vit. and Horm. 14, 187. New York: Academic Press. 1956.

Sieradzki, J., Schatz, H., Nierle, C., Pfeiffer, E. F., A possible role of glucagon in the mechanism of somatostatin-induced inhibition of insulin release. Diabetologia 11 (1975), 376.

Sirek, O. V., Hotta, N., Sirek, A., Acute metabolic effects of growth hormone and their relationship to insulin. Diabetes. Proc. 7th Congr. Internat. Diabetes Fed. p. 175. Amsterdam: Excerpta Medica. 1971.

Söling, H. D., Die Rolle der Leber im Kohlenhydratstoffwechsel des Organismus. Niedersächs. Ärzteblatt 47, Nr. 11 (1974), 416.

Sokal, J. E., Glucagon—an essential hormone. Am. J. Med. *41*, No. 3 (1966), 331.
— Sarcione, E. J., Henderson, A. M., The relative potency of glucagon and epinephrine as hepatic glycogenolytic agens: Studies with isolated perfused rat liver. Endocrin. *74* (1964), 930.
Soskin, S., Levine, R., Carbohydrate metabolism. Chicago, Ill.: The University of Chicago Press. 1952.
Spatz, H., Das Hypophysen-Hypothalamus-System in Hinsicht auf die zentrale Steuerung der Sexualfunktion. 1. Symp. Dtsch. Ges. Endokrin., S. 1—44. Berlin-Heidelberg-New York: Springer. 1955.
Stewart, G. N., Rogoff, J. M., The relation of the adrenals to piqûre hyperglycemia and to the glycogen content of the liver. Am. J. Physiol. *46* (1918), 90.
Stremmel, W., Untersuchungen zur Pathogenese des transitorischen Diabetes mellitus nach Operationen. Thesis Freiburg (Hab.-Schrift vom 12. Juli 1972).
— Die Bedeutung des Fettstoffwechsels bei chirurgischen Erkrankungen. Die Infusionstherapie *1*, Nr. 3 (1974), 238.
— Zur Pathogenese der Kohlenhydratstoffwechselstörungen nach operativen Eingriffen. Die Infusionstherapie *1*, Nr. 4 (1974), 294.
— Der Einfluß von Alpha-Rezeptorenblockern auf die stimulierende Insulinsekretion während Narkose und Operation. Die Infusionstherapie *1*, Nr. 4 (1974), 307.
— Kümmerle, H., Kruse-Jarres, J. D., The effect of Arginine infusion upon insulin secretion during intraabdominal operation. Diabetologia *11* (1975), 378.
Strieck, F., Beiträge zur Kenntnis der zentralnervösen Stoffwechselregulation. Verhandl. Dtsch. Ges. Nerv. Ärzte. 22. Jahresversammlg. S. 40—48. Berlin: F. C. W. Vogel. 1935.
— Experimenteller Beitrag zur Frage des zerebralen Diabetes. Z. Exper. Med. *104* (1938), 232.
Sutherland, E. W., Robinson, G. A., The role of cyclic AMP in the control of carbohydrate metabolism. Diabetologia *18* (1969), 797.
Szentàgothai, J., Nervale Schaltmechanismen der hypothalamo-hypophysären Steuerung. Verhandlg. Dtsch. Ges. Inn. Med. 71. Kongr. S. 42. München 1965.
Tausk, M., Pharmakologie der Hormone. Stuttgart: G. Thieme. 1973.
Unger, R. H., Glucagon and the insulin/glucagon ratio in diabetes and other catabolic illnesses. Diabetes *20*, No. 12 (1971), 834.
— Insulin/glucagon ratio. Israel. J. Med. Sci. *8* (1972), 252.
— persönliche Mitteilung (1975).
— Eisentraut, A. M., Entero-insular axis. Arch. Intern. Med. *123* (1969), 261.
— Aguilar-Parada, E., Muller, W. A., Eisentraut, A. M., Studies of pancreatic alpha-cell function in normal diabetic subjects. J. Clin. Invest. *49* (1970), 837.
— Faloona, G. R., The roles of pancreatic glucagon in health and diabetes mellitus. Diabetes. Proc. 7th Congr. Internat. Diabetes Fed. p. 601. Amsterdam: Excerpta Medica. 1971.
— Lefebvre, P., Glucagon physiology (Lefebvre, P., Unger, R. H., eds.), p. 213. New York-Toronto-Sydney-Braunschweig: Pergamon Press. 1972.
Vallance-Owen, J., Insulin antagonists and inhibitors. Advances in Metab. Disord. (Levine, R., Luft, R., eds.), Vol. 1, p. 191. New York-London: Academic Press. 1964.
Valle, J., Nauta, H., Haymaker, W., Hypothalamic nuclei and fiber connections. In: The hypothalamus, p. 136. Springfield, Ill.: Ch. C Thomas. 1969.
Van der Meer, C., Diagnostik des Hypothalamus-Hypophysen-Nebennierenrindensystems. In: ACTH — eine Standortbestimmung für die Praxis (Schuppli, R., Hrsg.), S. 19. Bern-Stuttgart: H. Huber. 1973.

Vasquez, A. M., Schutt-Aine, J., Drash, A. L., Kenny, F. M., Diurnal patterns of secretion of cortisol and growth hormone in normal adolescents, in patients with exogenous and endogenous Cushing's syndrome, in patients with diabetes mellitus, and in a fasting subject. Pediatrics *83*, No. 4 (1973), 578.

Veil, W. H., Sturm, A., Die Pathologie des Stammhirns. Jena: G. Fischer. 1952.

Vonderrahe, A. R., Central nervous system and sugar metabolism. Arch. Int. Med. *60* (1937), 694.

— Central nervous system and diabetes mellitus. Ohio Med. J. *33* (1937 a), 1315.

Walli, A. K., Schimassek, H., Regulation of carbohydrate metabolism. In: Modern aspects of neurosurgery (Pia, H. W., Grote, E., Mundinger, F., Gleave, J. R. W., eds.), Vol. 2, p. 182. Amsterdam: Excerpta Medica. 1971.

Watari, N., Fine structure of nervous elements in the pancreas of some vertebrates. Z. Zellforschung *85* (1968), 291.

Wedler, H. W., Zur Frage der zentralen Entstehung innerer Krankheiten. Verhandlg. Dtsch. Ges. Inn. Med. *54* (1948), 136.

Weissbecker, L., Regelprinzipien bei der adenohypophysären Inkretion und ihre Bedeutung. Verhandlg. Dtsch. Ges. Inn. Med. 71. Kongr. S. 71. München 1965.

Wesemann, W., personal report 1975.

— Grote, E., Diabetes mellitus and diabetes insipidus: a syndrome of hypothalamic dysregulation? In: Modern aspects of neurosurgery (Pia, H. W., Grote, E., Mundinger, F., Gleave, J. R. W., eds.), Vol. 2, p. 208. Amsterdam: Excerpta Medica. 1971.

— — Pia, H. W., Energy requirement and energy balance in patients with brain tumors and injuries. Internat. Congr. Ser. *293*, 84. Amsterdam-Princetown-London-Geneva-Tokyo: Excerpta Medica. 1973.

— — Hyperglykaemien: Verlaufsbeobachtungen bei Patienten mit zerebralen Tumoren und Verletzungen. In: Diabetes mellitus (Beringer, A., Hrsg.), S. 723. Wien-München-Bern: W. Maudrich. 1973.

Westermann, E., Stock, K., The autonomic nervous system and energy metabolism. J. Neuro-Visc. Rel. Suppl. *IX*, 283. Wien-New York: Springer. 1969.

Wicklmayr, M., Dietze, G., On the regulation of pyruvate oxidation in the human central nervous system (CNS) during fasting. Diabetologia *11* (1975), 383.

Wiegelmann, W., Wachstumshormon und Gonadotropine bei Erkrankungen des Hypothalamus-Hypophysensystems. München-Berlin-Wien: Urban & Schwarzenberg. 1973.

Wild, H., Simon, K., Die Bedeutung der verschiedenen Zuckerbelastungsproben für die Diagnose krankhafter Prozesse im Hypophysen-Zwischenhirnbereich. Zschr. klin. Med. *146* (1950), 644.

Wilder, J., Das „Ausgangswertgesetz", ein unbeachtetes biologisches Gesetz und seine Bedeutung für Forschung und Praxis. Ges. Neurol. Psych. *137* (1931), 317.

Willers, F. A., Methoden der praktischen Analysis. Berlin: W. de Gruyter & Co. 1957.

Williams, R. H., Porte, D., jr., The pancreas. In: Textbook of endocrinology (Williams, R. H., ed.). Philadelphia-London-Toronto: Saunders Congress. 1974.

Wilmore, D. W., Lindsey, C. A., Moyland, J. A., Faloona, G. R., Pruitt, B. A., Unger, R. H., Hyperglucagonemia after burns. Lancet *19* (1974), 73.

Winborn, W. B., Light and electron microscopy of the islets of Langerhans of the Saimiri monkey pancreas. Anatom. Rec. *147* (1963), 65.

Woods, S. C., Porte, D., jr., Neural control of the endocrine pancreas. Physiol. Rev. *54*, No. 3 (1974), 596.

Yalow, R. S., Berson, S. A., Secretory responses of HGH and ACTH in diabetic and non-diabetic subjects. Diabetes. Proc. 7th Congr. Internat. Diabetes Fed. S. 741. Amsterdam: Excerpta Medica. 1971.

Yamada, E., Some observations on the nerve terminal of the liver parenchymal cell of the mouse as revealed by electron microscopy. Okajimas Fol. Anat. Jap. *40* (1965), 663.

Zülch, H. J., Vegetative und psychische Symptome bei umschriebenen traumatischen Zwischenhirnschädigungen und ihre Beurteilung im Gutachten. Zentralblatt Neurochir. *10* (1950), 73.

Zunz, E., LaBarre, J., Sur l'augmentation de la teneur en insuline du sang veineux pancréatique. Compt. Rend. Soc. Biol. *96* (1927), 421.

— — Sur la sensibilité des centres nerveux supérieurs à l'hyperglycémie provoquée par injection de dextrose. Compt. Rend. Soc. Belge Biol. 1400 (1927).